Stressed Out

About the NCLEX-RN®

Patricia M. Pierce, ARNP, PhD, FAAN

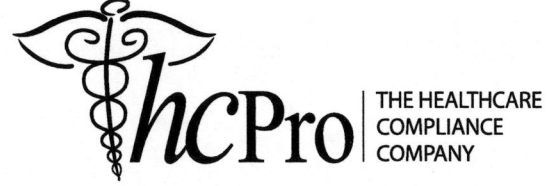

Stressed Out About the NCLEX-RN® by Patricia M. Pierce, ARNP, PhD, FAAN

Published by HCPro, Inc. Copyright ©2007 HCPro, Inc.

All rights reserved. Printed in the United States of America.   5 4 3 2 1

ISBN 978-1-57839-893-5

No part of this publication may be reproduced, in any form or by any means, without prior written consent of HCPro, Inc., or the Copyright Clearance Center (978/750-8400). Please notify us immediately if you have received an unauthorized copy.

HCPro, Inc., provides information resources for the healthcare industry.

HCPro, Inc., is not affiliated in any way with the Joint Commission on Accreditation of Healthcare Organizations, which owns the JCAHO trademark.

Patricia M. Pierce, ARNP, PhD, FAAN, Author
Rebecca Hendren, Managing Editor
Emily Sheahan, Group Publisher
Shane Katz, Cover Designer
Mike Mirabello, Senior Graphic Artist
Jean St. Pierre, Director of Operations
Darren Kelly, Production Coordinator
Audrey Doyle, Copyeditor

Cover illustration by Graham Smith, ArtMasters

Advice given is general. Readers should consult professional counsel for specific legal, ethical, or clinical questions.

Arrangements can be made for quantity discounts. For more information, contact

HCPro, Inc.
P.O. Box 1168
Marblehead, MA 01945
Telephone: 800/650-6787 or 781/639-1872
Fax: 781/639-2982
E-mail: *customerservice@hcpro.com*

Visit the *Stressed Out* Web site for more information: *www.stressedoutnurses.com*

Dedication

To my sons. Unique people with unique ideas.

Contents

How to use this book xi

About the author xiii

Introduction xv

Part 1: Preparation—What do I need to do?

Chapter 1: The final hurdle 3

    The NCLEX-RN® 3
    The exam of all exams 3
    If you made it through nursing school, you can do this 4
        Take a minute to relax 4

Chapter 2: The lowdown on paperwork 7

    How do I apply to take the NCLEX? 7
        Your nursing school's role 7
    It's all about safety 8
    Who administers the test? 8
    How do I get started? 9
    What do I send to Pearson VUE? 9
        Obtaining a sit pass 9
        Stay within the time frame 10

    Filling in the registration form 10
  How much money do I need? 11
    Is there help to pay for the NCLEX? 12
  Where is the test offered? 12

Chapter 3: Before the test 15

  Do questions test what I really need to know? 15
  What kind of questions should I expect? 16
  What should I bring to the exam? 16
    What should I wear to the exam? 17
  Confidentiality agreement 17

Chapter 4: The NCLEX mystery unveiled 19

  Test construction 19
  The NCLEX is a marathon, not a sprint 20
  How many questions are there? 20
    Why did I get 265 questions when my best friend got only 136? 21
  During my test... 22
  Is it like other tests I have taken? 22
  Calm your nerves with the practice tutorial 24
  What score do I need to pass? 24
    Results time 25
  After the test 25
  Real-life experiences 26
  It's all about you 26

Part 2: Question breakdown

Chapter 5: All about the questions 29

  The key to NCLEX is applying your learning 29
  The main focus of the NCLEX 30

Chapter 6: Safe and Effective Care Environment 33

    Management of Care subsection 33
    Safety and Infection Control subsection 38

Chapter 7: Health Promotion and Maintenance 43

Chapter 8: Psychosocial Integrity 47

Chapter 9: Physiological Integrity 53

    Basic Care and Comfort subsection 53
    Pharmacological and Parenteral Therapies subsection 56
    Reduction of Risk Potential subsection 59
    Physiological Adaptation subsection 62

Part 3: Studying—Making the most of your time

Chapter 10: Take a look at yourself—warts and all 67

    It's study time 67
        What should I do about my weak knowledge areas? 68
    The exam before the exam 68
    Study map for NCLEX preparation 70
    Study resources 72
        Textbooks 72
        Review courses 72
        The NCSBN 72
        The National League for Nursing 73
        Publications 73
        Kaplan and ATI 73
        Your college 74
        Online 74
    Practice makes perfect 75
    How I passed the NCLEX 75

Chapter 11: Develop a study plan 77

What don't you know? 77
Tips for successful studying: Have a plan 77
    Start with a study plan 78
    Don't procrastinate 79
    Find your zone 80
    Stick to a routine 80
    Prioritize 80
    Concentrate 80
    Change it up 80
    Friends with benefits 80
    Treat yourself 81

Chapter 12: Critical thinking and the NCLEX 85

Critical thinking: The pathway to success 85
    What is critical thinking? 85
    Do I have critical-thinking skills? 87
    Using critical thinking in the NCLEX 87

Chapter 13: Test-taking strategies 91

Reading the question 91
Understanding the question 93
    Practice 93
    English as a second language 94

Chapter 14: Choosing the right answer 95

How do I decide between two right answers? 95
    I'm still unsure 96
Should I guess? 97
Question dissection 97

Chapter 15: Topics for serious review 99

Basic areas for serious review 99
Laboratory values 101
    Making safe choices 102

Chapter 16: If they passed, so can you 105

I think I'm going to fail 105
    If more than a million people have passed, so can I 105
Pass rate breakdown 106

Part 4: Stress—How do you spell stress relief?

Chapter 17: Take a deep breath 111

How stressed are you? 114
Free, easy, and available now 115
Breathing: You have to do it, so why not do it right? 115
    Breathing under stress 116
    Take a deep breath 116
    It's good for you, too 117

Chapter 18: Exercise your stress away 119

The merit badge of exercise 119
Schedule your exercise 119
    Find a buddy 121
You put one foot in front of the other 122
    Walking and listening 122
Balance your body with yoga 123
What about tai chi? 124
Exercise without even noticing 124

Chapter 19: Manage stress by living well 127

- Meditation 128
  - Anyone can meditate 128
- Go to your happy place 129
- Eat for the NCLEX 129
- Avoid caffeine, alcohol, and cigarettes 131
- Don't let others drag you down 131
  - Just say no 132
- Don't forget to enjoy yourself 132

Chapter 20: The big day 135

- Relaxation techniques for the NCLEX 136
- During the test 137
- What worried you? 137
- What if I'm taking the test and I hit a snag? 138
  - Think about what you know 139
- You are ready! 140

Appendix

Study guide quiz 143

Resources 147

Glossary 155

References 159

Study guide quiz answers 161

How to use this book

What if there was a book that explained complex nursing topics in an easy-to-understand manner and in an accessible format? That's the premise behind the *Stressed Out...* series. Solid references with a bit of a sense of humor and the understanding that a lighthearted approach to learning makes the whole thing more enjoyable.

To help you navigate through the book, you will find the following icons highlighting a particular passage:

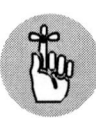

Don't forget: A little reminder about something of importance.

Ask: This icon directs you to search for further information from an individual or organization.

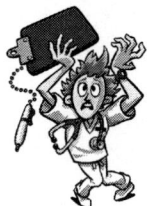

Don't panic: Take a deep breath and relax. Here is a little reassurance.

Fact: Highlights a statistic or truth.

 **Tip:** A bit of inside information, a hint, or helpful advice.

 **Watch out:** Word to the wise; this is a warning.

 **Click:** This icon refers you to a helpful Web Site, where you may find further information on the topic.

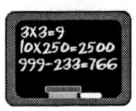 **Example:** Highlights sample questions and step-by-step solutions.

Happy Nursing! Now you're ready to get started.

About the author

Patricia M. Pierce, ARNP, PhD, FAAN

Dr. Patricia Pierce, ARNP, PhD, FAAN, has more than 25 years experience as a nurse educator. She is currently an educator at the Bay Pines VA Health Care System in St. Petersburg, FL, and is shared faculty to St. Petersburg College. During her long career in nursing education she has held faculty positions at the University of Texas, University of Florida, University of Tampa, St. Leo University, and the University of Phoenix.

Pierce serves as an appraiser for the American Nurses Credentialing Center's Magnet Recognition Program® and the *Tampa Bay Business Journal* recently nominated her as a "Health Care Hero" in its annual recognition program for educators. Her past experience includes positions as CEO of her own pediatric healthcare company, executive director of a large home care company, and an independent consultant for case management and healthcare legal issues. She has published frequently in journals and has been an invited speaker at numerous conferences.

Introduction

You made it through nursing school, but you still have to pass the NCLEX-RN® before you can finally begin your dream career. Right now, you're probably thinking, "How can I possibly remember all those things I learned in nursing school?"

Don't panic. Nursing school has armed you with all the information you need to succeed, and with some careful planning and a little help from this book, you can overcome your worries and prepare to take the test with confidence.

This book will guide you through:

- How the exam works, so you won't be freaked out by any surprises
- The application process and everything you need to prepare
- The ins and outs of analyzing questions
- Boosting your critical-thinking skills
- Techniques to manage your stress

Complete with advice and experiences from recent graduates who are NCLEX survivors, this book will guide you through your study period and prepare you for success.

Your nursing career awaits. Take a deep breath and dive in!

Part One

Before you can begin studying for the NCLEX, you probably want to know what it entails. This section explains how the test works, how to apply, and everything you need to know to prepare for the big day.

Chapter 1

The final hurdle

You did it! You passed all the tests, wrote all the care plans, used every therapeutic communication technique in the book, and made it through that brain-twisting end-of-program exit exam. You have just one more mountain to climb before you begin your exciting journey as a nurse . . .

The NCLEX-RN®!

And right now it probably feels like Everest itself is looming in front of you, with your hopes and dreams for your career waiting on the other side.

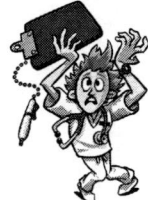

Don't panic: The mountain is *not* insurmountable. Listen to this: Just between January and September of 2006, 148,305 people passed the NCLEX (NCSBN 2006). That's a lot of people! And if they can do it, so can you.

The key is to study smart, be prepared, and above all, not get stressed out!

The exam of all exams

Fact: NCLEX stands for **N**ational **C**ouncil **L**icensure **Ex**amination, and it is designed to determine whether you can practice safely as a beginning practitioner. The same exam—with varying questions, of course—is given to every graduate of every nursing school. Yes, diploma, associate degree, and baccalaureate degree graduates all take the same exam for the same RN license.

Chapter 1   The final hurdle

The NCLEX is the final hurdle before you begin your nursing career, but once you have passed it, your career begins and you are free to soar as high as you want. You need to pass the NCLEX only once, and once you do, you are free to practice in any state in the country.

Although the NCLEX may seem arduous, today's takers actually have it better than in the past. In the old days of the NCLEX, the test lasted two full days and was divided into five parts, which covered medical nursing, surgical nursing, pediatrics, obstetrics, and psychiatry. These topics are now integrated into the NCLEX and the test is administered within a six-hour period.

If you made it through nursing school, you can do this

Regardless of whether you have recently graduated, are a final-year nurse, or have just started nursing school but are planning ahead, the important thing to remember is that you *can* pass the NCLEX. Before you get into panic mode, think about how successful you have been to get to this point. First, you had to be accepted into nursing school, which is a pretty tough achievement. You've also made it through grueling clinicals and tough classes. You have studied hard and packed hours of knowledge into your brain.

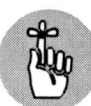

Don't forget: You *are* ready to be successful on the NCLEX. You *are* ready to be a valuable asset to the nursing profession.

Take a minute to relax

So, first things first: If you've just graduated, you may consider taking a quick breather before hitting the books. Here is what some soon-to-graduate seniors and a three-year veteran nurse have to say about their study plans and the period after graduation.

So decide if you want to do something to clear your mind and do it. Then refocus and get started. You *can* pass NCLEX, but only if you prepare. This book will walk you through the process. It will give you practical advice, test-taking skills, and ways to chase that stress away. Let's get started.

The final hurdle

> *"I just finished the final and end-of-program. I can't think about the NCLEX now. I have done well on tests, so I will study, but I'm not really worried."*
>
> —A.S., senior nursing student
>
> *"After I finish my 12-hour shift, I am too tired to think about studying. I'll begin after pinning. I have a study plan."*
>
> —J.T., senior nursing student
>
> *"I feel as if what I am learning in this practicum is studying, so I put the books down for a while."*
>
> —C.B., senior nursing student
>
> *"Right after pinning, I jumped on a plane and took a two-week vacation."*
>
> —R.C., three-year veteran nurse

References

NCSBN. 2006. *NCLEX Statistics from NCSBN*. Available at *www.ncsbn.org*.

Chapter 2

The lowdown on paperwork

How do I apply to take the NCLEX?

Okay, let's begin at the beginning. Before you can take the exam, you have to apply. You must fill out the application forms correctly and send everything, along with the correct amount of money, to the right place. The fee for the licensure exam varies by state, so check with the Board of Nursing in your state to find out how much it will cost you. You need to know the exact amount to be sure your application does not get delayed because you sent insufficient funds.

Your nursing school's role

Fact: Your school of nursing submits the list of students who have successfully completed all the requirements for graduation to the State Board of Nursing. The school sends the list to the state where the school is located—if you want to take the board in a different state, you must have the school send record of your eligibility to that state.

The school also verifies that your coursework met the requirements for any continuing education units mandated by the State Board of Nursing. For example, some, but not all, states require a certain number of hours spent learning about HIV-AIDS, domestic violence, or medical errors. Your school guarantees that your curriculum contained the necessary information and met all the requirements.

It's all about safety

The Board of Nursing in your state is a member of the National Council of State Boards of Nursing (NCSBN), which has a mandate to protect the public's health, safety, and welfare. The NCSBN does this by making sure that nurses who are licensed have achieved at least a minimum level of knowledge and skill. And it does that by administering the NCLEX, a standardized bank of test questions specifically designed to ensure that test takers are competent to practice at a beginning level.

Many states now require a criminal background check before candidates are deemed eligible to sit for the NCLEX. If your state requires a criminal background check, the fee for it is covered by your licensing application fee.

Watch out: A word to the wise about the background check: If you have ever been convicted of a crime, or if you have ever entered a guilty plea or a *nolo contendere* plea, be sure to share that information with the state board. Each applicant's situation is reviewed on a case-by-case basis and the board will consider the nature, severity, and recency of the offense.

Many schools of nursing already perform a background check when students first enter a nursing program. The schools are trying to prevent someone from finishing the school requirements but then being deemed ineligible for the state board. If you have any questions about this part of the application, contact your school advisor and your state board.

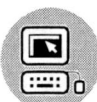

Click: You can find a complete listing of which states require background checks at the NCSBN Web site, *www.ncsbn.org*.

Who administers the test?

Fact: The NCLEX is administered by Pearson VUE, a company focused on electronic testing and dedicated to the professional licensure and certification market. VUE stands for **V**irtual **U**niversity **E**nterprises and the company is an international testing resource for many professions.

The NCLEX is a computer-based exam, which means you can only take it at specific venues where the computer is installed. These venues are test centers approved by Pearson VUE. Pearson provides the testing site and verifies that applicants are who they say they are. Pearson provides camera surveillance during the testing period and sends your computer results to the board.

How do I get started?

Remember that the registration process involves several steps and you need to complete each step correctly before you can receive an accurate ticket to take to the test center as your admittance to the NCLEX. As noted earlier, your first step is to send an application to the state board.

The applications for the state board or territory where you plan to be licensed are available online. Make sure the application is filled out completely. Enclose the correct amount of money in the form of a cashier's check, certified check, money order, or credit card verification. If you apply online, you must pay by credit card: Visa, MasterCard, or American Express.

What do I send to Pearson VUE?

Watch out: Applicants planning to take the NCLEX have to fill in two application forms and pay two application fees. As noted earlier, you send one application form to your state board. You send the other application form (called a *registration*) to Pearson VUE. You can send both applications electronically or by U.S. mail. To apply electronically, you must have a valid credit card. Most applicants find it easier to send both applications at the same time.

Although the fee that accompanies the application you send to the state board varies by state, the fee that accompanies the registration you send to Pearson is $200, and that fee must accompany the application. You can pay by money order, certified check, cashier's check, Visa, MasterCard, or American Express.

Click: If you have questions about the process, you can visit the NCLEX Candidate Web Site at *www.pearsonvue.com/nclex*. Or call 1-866-49NCLEX (1-866/496-2539).

Obtaining a sit pass

After you register with Pearson VUE to take the exam and the state board has confirmed that you are eligible, Pearson will issue your Authorization to Test (ATT), commonly referred to as a "sit pass." Without the ATT, you cannot schedule an appointment to take the exam.

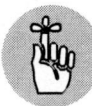

Don't forget: You *must* present the ATT at the examination site in order to be admitted.

Click: You can find a complete list of national and international test centers, along with the Pearson registration form, at *www.pearsonvue.com/nclex*.

Stay within the time frame

Watch out: You must test during the time frame specified on your ATT and these times may vary by state. Most ATTs are valid for 90 days and you must request an appointment within that time frame, but pay attention to the time frame for your ATT. Pearson *does not* extend the dates for any reason (Candidate Bulletin 2006).

Your eligibility from the State Board of Nursing is good for 365 days, so you need to pay most attention to the Pearson time frame. Don't send in your registration until you are ready. Many students do send both applications at the same time, but you could wait a few days after applying to the State Board to give the Board time to update records if you are concerned about meeting the 90 day time period.

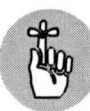

Don't forget: In addition to the ATT, you must present acceptable photo identification when you arrive for your test. Acceptable identification includes a passport, valid driver's license, state identification, national identity card, or U.S. military ID with visible signature. Note that learner's permits are *not* accepted.

If you will require special accommodations during the test you must submit your request to your state board of nursing and the NCSBN before you submit your registration form to Pearson. The procedure for requesting special accommodations is explained in the Candidate Bulletin.

Filling in the registration form

You may register with Pearson VUE either online or via U.S. mail and you must fill in the registration form completely and correctly. Be sure to indicate whether you are taking the RN or the PN exam. If you choose the wrong one and you need to change it, there is a $50 change fee.

Watch out: Here are some words of caution to anyone who gets married or divorced between graduation and the NCLEX. Be sure the name on your registration is exactly the same as the one on the identification you will take with you in order to enter the examination. If you applied before you got married, don't change the name on your picture ID until *after* you take the NCLEX. Your mother's maiden name (the name she had when she was born) is also used as a security check. The phone number you list as your home or mobile number is the one Pearson will use if it needs to contact you about your registration.

When filling in the registration form, fill in the blanks with the correct letters or numbers and blacken the corresponding circles. Don't leave anything blank because doing so will delay the registration process. Take your time, stay focused, and be accurate. This will probably remind you of the scantrons you completed for tests in nursing school.

If you provide an e-mail address when you register, all your correspondence from Pearson VUE will arrive *only* via e-mail. If you do not provide an e-mail address when you register, your correspondence will arrive *only* via U.S. mail.

You should receive confirmation and your ATT from Pearson VUE within two weeks of registering. If you do not receive these items, contact Pearson VUE via telephone. People are available to talk with you Monday through Friday, from 7 a.m. until 7 p.m. Central time, at 866/496-2539. Do not send another registration without calling first to check on the status of your application.

A word to the wise: This service has been outsourced, so make sure you have all the information you need, such as your name as it appears on your registration, your mother's maiden name, and so on, with you when you call to expedite the process (Candidate Bulletin 2006).

Need help filling out the form?

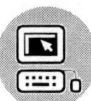

A good first step is to visit the NCSBN Web site, at *www.ncsbn.org*, and print out the NCLEX Examination Candidate Bulletin. The bulletin provides a detailed explanation of how to complete the application process.

How much money do I need?

How much money you need varies from state to state. The fee charged by Pearson to take the NCLEX is $200 in every state, however, some state boards have additional fees. Check with your board to determine whether any additional fees are applicable in the state or territory where you are testing. An additional $150 is charged to candidates who request to take the exam at an international testing site. Neither of these fees is refunded if the candidate does not take the exam within the 365-day time frame for the Board of Nursing or the 90-day time frame once you receive your ATT.

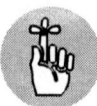

Don't forget: Once you receive your ATT, the time you have to take the exam is determined by the dates on the ATT. Once again, Pearson does not extend these dates.

Remember, you may pay for the examination via credit card if you're registering online or over the telephone. Only Visa, MasterCard, and American Express are accepted. To pay by check, you must have a cashier's check, money order, or certified check—personal checks are not accepted.

Is there help to pay for the NCLEX?

Some counties and states have funds available for candidates who cannot afford the application fees. Check with your state board of nursing, school of nursing, and county work programs.

Some areas also offer work net programs that assist low-income applicants as part of the Federal Welfare-to-Work Hiring Initiative. Your school's financial aid office may also have some resources you can try.

Some hospitals may even pay for the NCLEX as a recruitment enticement to get you to agree to a job with that organization. So, if you are interviewing, ask whether paying for the NCLEX is part of the package. Keep in mind, however, that many hospitals will expect you to pass on the first try and may even dismiss employees who are not successful.

Where is the test offered?

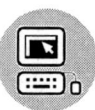

Click: Pearson VUE has numerous test centers throughout the United States and in many foreign countries. For a complete list of centers, visit the Pearson VUE Web site, at *www.pearsonvue.com/nclex*.

First-time test takers are usually able to take the exam within 30 days of applying. Repeat takers usually are seated within 45 days.

Tip: Seats are limited and they fill up quickly, so schedule your exam as soon as you receive your ATT.

Some applicants have reported delays in availability, or the need to travel to alternative sites, to schedule the NCLEX in a timely manner. So, if your area has many graduates at the time you are graduating, be prudent and apply as early as possible. Statistics have shown that those who take the test within 30 days after graduation do significantly better than those who delay taking the NCLEX.

Application process at a glance

1. Submit an application for licensure to the Board of Nursing in the state or territory where you wish to be licensed.

2. Register for the NCLEX examination with Pearson VUE.

3. Receive confirmation of registration from Pearson VUE.

4. The Board of Nursing verifies that the candidate is eligible to take the NCLEX.

5. You will receive an Authorization to Test (ATT) from Pearson VUE.

6. Contact Pearson to schedule the date and time of your exam.

References

National Council of State Boards of Nursing. (2006). *2006 Candidate Bulletin*. Page 8. Available at *https://www.ncsbn.org/2006_Candidate_Bulletin.pdf*.

Chapter 3

Before the test

Do questions test what I really need to know?

Nursing profession experts apply to the National Council of State Boards of Nursing (NCSBN) to write the NCLEX test questions. Many test writers are faculty members at associate degree and baccalaureate nursing programs. All questions are reviewed by an expert panel to ensure that they are appropriate for entry-level nurses. No items are used in a test without first being pretested and found statistically sound.

The test writers are constantly writing new questions to keep the test relevant and to ensure that it is an appropriate assessment of what new nurses need to know. Each year, new trial questions are added to the NCLEX for possible inclusion in the following year's test. These new questions are embedded in each test so that the NCSBN can gather information about their difficulty and validity. They are not counted as part of the test taker's score and there is no way for you to tell whether a question is new and is being tested for difficulty and validity.

The NCSBN conducts ongoing analysis of nursing practice, client needs, and key issues in safety for those receiving nursing care to determine what questions will be asked on the test. In addition to including questions related to fundamental knowledge for nurses, the test plan reflects key aspects of current practice.

What kind of questions should I expect?

Fact: The test writers develop the test around a predetermined plan that incorporates both the art and the science of nursing and is based on the belief that nursing integrates knowledge from many disciplines, including biology, physiology, psychology, and social science. The overarching design is based on the philosophy that the goal of nursing is "to prevent illness; alleviate suffering; and protect, promote, and restore health" (NCLEX Test Plan 2004).

Using Bloom's taxonomy, most questions require application of knowledge, skills, abilities, and complex cognitive processes. You probably remember hearing about Benjamin S. Bloom in nursing school. Bloom was an educator who designed a method for classifying learning and testing according to difficulty. He determined that application of knowledge was the highest order of learning, so it will come as no surprise that almost all the questions on the NCLEX are application-of-knowledge questions.

The test plan includes a variety of test question styles. Standard multiple choice questions are the mainstay of the exam. However, the test also includes fill-in-the-blank questions, questions that ask candidates to "select all that apply," and those that require math calculations (an online calculator is provided during the test). Another type of question presents a drawing or picture and requires the candidate to answer the question by pointing to and clicking the specific place on the picture that answers the question.

What should I bring to the exam?

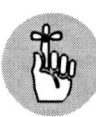

Don't forget: You must bring your Authorization to Test (ATT) and picture identification because you will not be admitted without them. And remember that the identification you bring must match the name on your ATT exactly. If your name has legally changed since you received your ATT, you must bring legal documentation to the test center (e.g., a marriage license, divorce decree, or legal court action). Be prepared to sign your name, be photographed, and be fingerprinted at the test center.

No one, including your children, is allowed in the test center with you. You must leave all of your personal belongings in the secure storage provided by the test center. Absolutely no nursing books or notebooks are permitted at the test center.

Each test center has a test administrator who provides you with a brief orientation and an erasable note board, and escorts you to a computer terminal. The test administrator is also available to help if you have problems with the computer. You have up to six hours to complete the exam. During this time you can take a short tutorial that demonstrates how the test works. You may take two optional breaks during the test.

Tip: Arrive early so that you do not feel rushed.

What should I wear to the exam?
Casual clothes you are physically comfortable wearing are best. You might want to layer, in case it is chilly in the test center. No hats, scarves, or coats are allowed in the testing room. Remember that security is a key issue for this test. If you tend to get cold, wear a long-sleeved shirt (you can always roll up the sleeves if necessary).

Confidentiality agreement

All candidates are required to sign a confidentiality agreement before leaving the testing room. Any violation of this agreement can lead to disciplinary action including civil liability and denial of licensure. This means you are on your honor not to share any questions you had on the test.

References

National Council of State Boards of Nursing (2004). *NCLEX Test Plan 2004*, p. 2. Available at *https://www.ncsbn.org/454.htm*.

Chapter 4

The NCLEX mystery unveiled

So how does this thing work and what are you going to find on the big day?

Test construction

Fact: A really nice aspect of the NCLEX is that every person who takes it receives a different exam. The NCLEX you take will be a unique test that is derived from a bank of more than 10,000 test questions.

Each question in the bank has been "tested" many times for difficulty and validity, so you can be sure the version of the NCLEX you receive is fair and comparable to every other version.

The National Council of State Boards of Nursing (NCSBN) constantly recruits test-question writers to ensure that the test bank remains current with contemporary nursing practice. If by some chance you are not successful, none of the questions you received will reappear on any subsequent test you take for at least one year. With 10,000 questions to choose from, the versions of the test are virtually endless.

The NCLEX uses Computer Adaptive Testing (CAT) to test all applicants. You may be asked as few as 75 questions or as many as 265 questions during the test.

Chapter 4 — The NCLEX mystery unveiled

The NCLEX is a marathon, not a sprint

The NCLEX is both similar to and different from every test you have taken in nursing school. It's similar because the format comprises mostly multiple choice questions in which you must select the best answer. It's different in that so much is riding on it.

It is computer-based and timed, and every NCLEX is unique; no two candidates receive exactly the same test. You will not know how many questions you will have to answer until you are finished. So pace yourself as though you expect to have to answer all 265 questions so that you won't run out of time.

Watch out: You have only one opportunity to answer a question. You cannot go back to a question if you suddenly figure out the correct answer later on during the test.

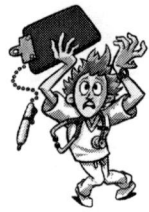

Don't panic: As the test progresses, you may receive questions that are similar to some you have already answered. Do not assume this means you answered the earlier questions incorrectly, and do not change your answers on the later questions to match those you provided for the earlier ones. These similar questions may be either new test questions (as discussed in Chapter 3) or just coincidentally similar to each other. In other words, for each question, always select the answer you believe to be correct.

The NCLEX's CAT format is designed to increase the difficulty of the questions you receive as the test progresses. Let's say you get a pediatric question about growth and development. If you answer it correctly your next question will be more complex and difficult, but if you answer it incorrectly you will receive another question at that level of complexity. In this way the test measures your level of competence. The Board is able to determine your knowledge and skill by using a formula that mixes topics with complexity and difficulty.

How many questions are there?

You will be required to answer at least 75 questions and at most 265 questions. You must answer every question presented to you because the computer does not allow you to proceed to the next question until you have chosen an answer for the current one.

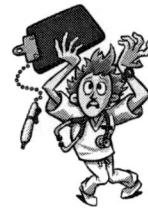

Don't panic: Seventy-five questions may be all it takes for the computer to determine your level of competence. But answering only 75 questions does not guarantee you passed—just as answering 265 questions does not mean you have failed. The computer keeps going until it has accurately measured your competence—and then the test ends.

Questions for your test are selected from the test bank of hundreds of questions and only your performance will determine how many questions your test will contain. A certain number of questions are required, and after that, testing ends when it can be determined, with a certainty of 95%, that you are either above or below the passing standard.

The test has been designed so that it is neither too hard nor too easy. It is intended to ensure that you are meeting the minimum standard of competency to become an RN. The NCSBN requires that you answer questions of a certain level of difficulty in order to continue with the test, to make certain that those who pass are competent to go on to provide patient care.

Approximately 15 of the items on your test will be "pretest" items that are not scored and do not count as part of your test. They are being "tested" for reliability and suitability for possible inclusion in tests for subsequent years. These items are analyzed statistically to determine whether they should be incorporated into the test bank. These 15 items are not part of your score, but you will not know when you are answering one of these questions.

Why did I get 265 questions when my best friend got only 136?

Your NCLEX test ends for the following reasons:

- You have answered 75 or more questions and have met the approved minimum competency.
- After answering 75 questions, you have not demonstrated the minimum level of competency.
- You have answered the maximum 265 questions.
- You have run out of time (six hours).

You may get any number of questions on your test. Just remember that the test shuts down when there is enough information to determine whether you have or have not demonstrated the minimal level of competency.

During my test...

Test experiences vary and you should not allow the test to make you panic.

> "I freaked out when the computer shut off after only 75 questions. I was sure I had answered only about 20 correctly. It turns out I passed."
>
> —T.F., recent graduate
>
> "I had trouble taking tests throughout nursing school. I braced myself for failure, because the test seemed so hard. But I passed the first time I took it!"
>
> —K.S., recent graduate
>
> "I was afraid I was going too slowly because I spent 3 hours on the first 81 questions. But, turns out that was all I needed to answer and PASS!"
>
> —J.M., recent graduate
>
> "I ended up only having to answer 95 questions. But I paced myself as if I would have to answer all 265."
>
> —I.M., recent graduate

Is it like other tests I have taken?

The NCLEX combines multiple choice questions with several variations. For example, some questions will tell you to "select all that apply," meaning that more than one answer may be correct. You must choose every correct response to receive credit for that question. But beware: It is possible that only one of the answers is correct. These questions require that you are able to discern between applicable and non-applicable choices based on the situation being presented in the question. These questions really call on your critical-thinking skills.

The NCLEX also includes quasi-interactive "point and click" types of questions. For these questions, you must locate the correct item on the screen and click it. For instance, the question may ask you to locate where you would listen for S2, or identify where the traction is incorrect. If you click the correct site, you receive credit for that question.

Short-answer questions have also been added to the NCLEX format. An example of a short-answer question is below. The example is from the NCLEX Test Review Web site, which was created by an RN who wants to help others prepare for the test.

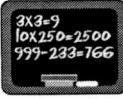

Example: RhoGAM is most often used to treat _____ mothers that have a _____ infant.

    a. RH positive, RH positive

    b. RH positive, RH negative

    c. RH negative, RH positive

    d. RH negative, RH negative

(The correct answer is c.)

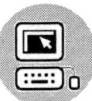

Click: You can find more examples of this type of question on the Web site, *www.nclexinfo.com.*

The NCLEX also includes math questions, and may require you to calculate a dose or figure the intake for a patient. The test computer has a calculator for your use.

Tip: Take your time with math questions. Be sure you are clear about what each question wants you to calculate.

The final category of questions comprises multiple choice options, and most of the questions you receive will be of this variety. You can count on every multiple choice question having at least two correct answers in the list of choices, and often, all of the responses to a particular question are correct. However, to receive credit for an answer in a multiple choice question, you must select the "best" answer.

For example, the stem of the question may ask you what you would do *first* in a certain situation, or which intervention has priority over the others, even though all the interventions are applicable in the given patient situation. You must select the "best" answer in order to receive credit for the answer.

Later, in Chapters 13 and 14, you will learn how to dissect questions so that you can make a thoughtful choice.

Calm your nerves with the practice tutorial

A brief tutorial is available for you to take before you begin the test. It provides you with a glimpse of the format of the test and is a good warm-up. You need not take it, but it takes only a few minutes to complete and may be a confidence builder to get you past the initial "stage fright" of the test itself. The tutorial is counted as part of your test time.

Tip: Test experts recommend that you complete the tutorial; it is very short and provides you with a clear description of the test process. Take it—it will help.

What score do I need to pass?

The criterion for passing the NCLEX is whether your answers indicate you have the knowledge and skill to perform at the "minimum level of ability required for safe and effective entry-level nursing practice" (NCSBN 2006).

The NCSBN Board of Directors sets the standard by gathering information from various sources. They use experts in psychometrics to evaluate how many correct answers reflect the standard. They review compiled historical data that contains comparisons of aggregate candidates' scores along with summaries of how candidates perform on the NCLEX. They solicit feedback from educators and employers to determine how well students perform in the clinical setting. They also examine how "educationally ready" the incoming pool of high school graduates is. By compiling information from many sources, the NCSBN is confident that the passing standard fulfills its obligation to ensure the public's health and safety.

Questions on the NCLEX are rated as "most difficult" and "easiest." No candidate is given all "most difficult" or all "easiest" questions. The extremes determine the point at which the candidate answers 50% of the questions correctly. The CAT program can then determine whether the candidate meets the expectation of achieving at least a 95% certainty for a minimum passing score.

Results time

Your score will not be available at the test center, so don't waste your time pleading with the staff of the center. The state board will send your results to you, and it usually takes anywhere from two weeks to a month.

Tip: Most state boards charge a small fee so that you can get your results about 48 hours after you take the test. If you can't wait, it may be worth the expense.

After the test

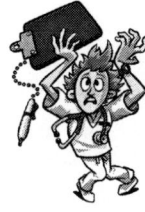

Don't panic: Almost everyone walking out of the test thinks they failed. If you only received 75 questions before the exam shut off, you may think you blew it, and if you received 265 questions before the exam ended, you also may think you blew it.

Real-life experiences

Look at what these recent candidates experienced.

> "My cell phone rang right after the test. It was someone inquiring about hiring me to tile a floor, a job I used to do before entering nursing school. I had not had such a call in two years and took it to be a very bad omen. I passed the NCLEX, however, and am now happily practicing as an RN, not a floor tiler."
>
> —S.G., RN
>
> "I received the maximum 265 questions and was so convinced I had failed that I actually began planning other ways to make a living. But I passed and am now happily practicing as an RN."
>
> —I.S., RN
>
> "I was so sure I had only answered about five questions correctly. Yet I must have done much better than that, because I passed."
>
> —J.D., RN
>
> "I walked out already thinking about the schedule for when I could repeat, until I found out I passed!"
>
> —E.Z., RN

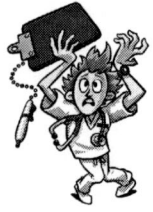

Don't panic: The moral of the story is to not jump to any conclusions. You will not know how well you did until you receive your results. There is no point beating yourself up. Just relax and wait for your results. For a small fee, you can receive your results in about 48 hours, or you can wait. The waiting may feel like an eternity, but try to relax and take your mind off the test for a short while.

It's all about you

The NCLEX is a comprehensive snapshot of what you know and how well you can apply your knowledge to difficult patient care situations. Remember that going into the test well prepared and confident will give you the edge you need to be successful. The next section will offer suggestions on ways to prepare for taking the NCLEX.

Part Two

When you are facing the NCLEX, it can be difficult to know where to start. This section walks you through the make-up of the questions and what you will be expected to know.

Chapter 5

All about the questions

The key to NCLEX is applying your learning

This section contains a detailed breakdown of the components of the NCLEX, and is intended to provide you with a broad approach to your preparation. You have learned so much throughout your time in nursing school and it is human nature to forget things, especially the material you learned early on in your nursing school career.

Remember, none of the questions you may be asked will simply test your knowledge. For example, you won't be given a blood gas and be asked what it represents. Instead, you may be asked to identify which nursing intervention should be done first.

Tip: When you are reading through the categories of questions in this section, keep in mind that questions will integrate concepts and information from more than one category of the test plan so that the candidate will have to analyze, prioritize, synthesize, and make decisions about complex patient situations. Further, knowledge of other disciplines, such as biology, sociology, growth, and development, will be needed to answer these complex questions.

You will not find any simple knowledge questions asking you to define a term. Rather, you will be tested on how you apply complex information to solve complex patient problems. Questions about critical care situations, disease management, and expected outcomes will be the rule of thumb.

The main focus of the NCLEX

The NCLEX is centered on key nursing practice areas and concerns. Although the percentage of questions in each area may vary in any given year, the focus areas remain stable. In keeping with the philosophy of nursing, areas of client need form the basis for the key areas. In every area of the NCLEX, candidates are expected to integrate knowledge from other disciplines and to apply knowledge of biological and social sciences.

The following box highlights the current test plan, which is the content areas for the NCLEX, and the percentage of questions dedicated to each area. These categories are basic nursing areas and the percentages do not vary much, if at all, from year to year. The topics are the same year to year, although in April 2007 questions about ergonomics will be added. The information is from the NCSBN Web site.

NCLEX test plan

NCLEX–RN® client areas 2004	% of items
Safe and Effective Care Environment	
Management of Care	13–19
Safety and Infection Control	8–14
Health Promotion and Maintenance	6–12
Psychosocial Integrity	6–12
Physiological Integrity	
Basic Care and Comfort	6–12
Pharmacological and Parenteral Therapies	13–19
Reduction of Risk Potential	13–19
Physiological Adaptation	11–17

As mentioned above, from April 2007 the NCLEX will include a section on ergonomics and its principles. This section is being added to emphasize the importance of safe patient handling to prevent injuries to both patients and nurses.

The rest of the chapters in this section focus on the four main areas of the NCLEX test plan. Chapters 6 to 9 discuss the categories of questions you can expect on the exam, along with subtopics within those categories. Also included are some key points that exemplify the kind of content you can expect to encounter within each of the areas from the test plan blueprint.

Watch out: Just as your tests in nursing school combined multiple aspects of a client's care, the NCLEX expects you to incorporate more than one approach when determining nursing interventions.

For example, a question may ask you to select the best health promotion teaching strategy for a client with end stage renal disease. To respond to a question like that, you must be able to integrate pharmacologic considerations with physiological aspects including safety, and so on.

So don't expect the questions to address just one part of the test plan at a time. The NCLEX expects you to use critical thinking skills to join many facets of care as you select your answer.

Reference

National Council of State Boards of Nursing. (2003). *Detailed Test Plan for the NCLEX-RN Examination.*

Chapter 6

Safe and Effective Care Environment

The first category in the NCLEX test plan is the Safe and Effective Care Environment category. Test questions included in this category focus on enhancing the healthcare environment to protect patients, family members, and healthcare personnel. This category of the test is divided into two subsections: Management of Care, and Safety and Infection Control.

Management of Care subsection

This subsection includes questions about enhancing client care, such as prioritizing your nursing actions and knowing when and what to delegate, as well as to whom you may delegate. Legal and ethical aspects of practice are also included, along with advocacy, case management, resource management, and client rights.

Specific examples of the kind of content areas you might receive are listed in the box that follows. Topics may include developing a user-friendly system that encourages staff to comply with a policy, or identifying when staff require more training regarding confidentiality.

Additional questions included under Management of Care cover topics such as staff education and supervision. These questions focus on the nurse as the manager of care for clients and families. For example, a question may concern a nurse who discovers that coworkers inconsistently follow the policy for verifying patient identification when administering medications. What actions could a staff nurse take to correct this behavior?

Management of Care

Following are key content areas from the detailed test plan within this subsection, with examples of what you may be asked:

Advance directives

- Be able to include information from other disciplines such as psychology or social work when involved in discussing advance directives with clients and their families/significant others.

- It is nurses' responsibility to incorporate the client's advance directive wishes into the overall plan of care.

Confidentiality

- Be responsible for maintaining patient confidentiality and seeing to it that other staff are adhering to the rules regarding patient information.

Multidisciplinary team collaboration

- Nurses must have in-depth knowledge of pathophysiology in order to be effective when collaborating with a multidisciplinary team.

- Nurses serve as client advocates and must be aware of circumstances that require input from other disciplines.

- Nurses sometimes feel as if their input is not as valuable as that of other disciplines. However, the nurse is the one who knows the client best and has valuable information that can improve care and outcomes.

Management of Care (cont.)

Continuity of care

- To ensure that the client receives "seamless" care, nurses must coordinate admissions and transfers so that accurate information is relayed to future caregivers.

- Nursing team members must give and receive accurate client information in order for care to address the needs of the client in a competent and timely manner.

- Nurses are responsible for discharge planning through collaborating with the interdisciplinary team and by providing patient and family education.

Establishing priorities

- Nurses must know how to perform those procedures routinely used in their practice area and must know when a different level of expertise is necessary to care for the client competently and safely.

- Whether working in the emergency department, long-term care, or general medical-surgical units, nurses must be able to prioritize care for a group of patients.

- Regardless of whether the care is emergent or routine, nurses must be able to prioritize care to address the needs of a group of clients.

Concepts of management

- Nurses must be able to relay information to colleagues so that care can continue effectively throughout all shifts.

- Nurses must be skilled communicators and able to use conflict resolution and problem-solving skills in a variety of situations, including with clients, families, and coworkers.

Management of Care (cont.)

- Nurses in management roles must be able to adapt clinical critical-thinking skills to the management arena.

Informed consent

- Nurses serve as client advocates to ensure that informed consent is obtained within the guidelines of professional nursing.

- Nurses serve as witnesses to acknowledge that clients sign the informed consent.

Legal rights and responsibilities

- Nurses must be familiar with legal issues surrounding client and family decisions, e.g., refusing certain interventions.

- Nurses cannot ignore unsafe practice and are responsible for making sure that those using unsafe practices are informed about proper techniques.

Performance improvement

- Nurses are responsible for recognizing when problems with a client's care require intervention from another team member, i.e., charge nurse, clinical specialist, risk manager.

- Nurses are expected to use current research to guide practice.

Referrals

- Nurses are expected to be familiar with community resources that can assist clients and their families.

- Nurses are expected to know how to initiate referrals to community and other resources.

Management of Care (cont.)

Staff education

- Rather than merely attending staff development activities, nurses are expected to be able to evaluate if the development activity was effective to improve practice.

Supervision

- Nurses are expected to oversee care given by nursing assistants and practical nurses to determine if the care was appropriately provided.

- Registered nurses are expected to recognize when other team members need assistance with time-management skills.

- The role of supervisor requires nurses to apply good critical-thinking skills.

Many of these topics were integrated throughout your nursing school curriculum. Don't overlook these nonphysiological areas. Recent NCLEX takers say they had many questions asking them to prioritize their nursing actions depending on the client's condition. Others say that questions concerning delegation appeared on their tests.

> *"I must have had eight or ten questions that asked me about delegating care to LPNs and NAs. I didn't expect so many about that."*
>
> —J.L., recent graduate
>
> *"I am so glad we had to learn how to prioritize patient care. I had several questions that asked about whom to care for first."*
>
> —D.R., recent graduate

Safety and Infection Control subsection

Safety and infection control are major concerns in contemporary hospitals. Some of the questions you can expect to receive in this area concern delegation, preventing medication errors and falls, and managing potential or real infection issues. Disaster planning and emergency management are also included, along with injury prevention in the hospital and at home. You are expected to know how to report an incident or variance in care, when and how to use restraints, and aseptic techniques.

With all of the recent emphasis on terrorism and natural disasters, applicants can expect to be asked about bioterrorism, first responders to a disaster, and triage priorities in a disaster situation. Questions in this subsection may ask about disaster planning and emergency response medications related to bioterrorism and the crash cart.

Know about safe communication techniques and accurate patient identification, particularly for high-risk interventions, such as blood administration, telephone orders, and surgery. Restraints and safety devices are also part of this subsection. Questions about protecting staff and patients from hazardous materials are directly related to safety.

Look for application questions that presume you know how to manage various isolation scenarios. They won't be as simple as asking what precautions you should take for a certain type of infection, but rather will expect you to apply what you know about infection control to a complex patient care situation.

Safe and Effective Care Environment — Chapter 6

Safety and Infection Control

Following are the key content areas included under the Safety and Infection Control subsection of the exam, with examples of what you may be asked:

Accident prevention

- Nurses are expected to prevent falls and other incidents by pre-emptively identifying clients with diminished sensory perception, i.e., vision, hearing loss.

- Nurses are expected to recognize how developmental level, age, and cognitive awareness can lead to accidents so that preventive measure can be implemented before something happens.

Handling hazardous and infectious materials

- Nurses must be able to apply standards of infection control to prevent the spread of infections.

- Nurses are expected to know how to identify hazardous materials and they should be familiar with where to find information about hazardous materials.

Home safety

- Clients and families should be involved in evaluating their environment and determining changes they can make to improve their safety.

- Nurses are expected to recognize safety hazards in the client's environment and to alter the environment to remove the hazard.

Injury prevention

- Nurses are expected to teach clients how to use protective equipment if they must use a potentially hazardous device for their care, i.e., disposal of syringes.

Safety and Infection Control (cont.)

- Nurses must recognize and remove fire hazards from the client's environment and be able to implement the agency fire safety procedures.

Medical and surgical asepsis

- Nurses must be able to identify and remove sources of infection from client care areas.

- Nurses must know how to use aseptic technique and must be able to evaluate if the technique has been followed appropriately.

Reporting of incident/event/irregular occurrence/variance

- As representatives of the employing agency and as client advocates, nurses are responsible for knowing when an incident report is required, i.e., client fall, wrong medication administered.

Safe use of equipment

- It is the nurse's responsibility to be sure any equipment used with a client is in good working order.

- Nurses are expected to use good judgment and know agency procedure in matters involving security.

Use of restraints/safety devices

- Nurses must be thoroughly familiar with agency policy and the Joint Commission for the Accreditation of Health Care Organizations' standards on use of restraint, as the inappropriate use of restraints can be considered false imprisonment.

- Whenever it is necessary to restrain a client, nurses are responsible for monitoring the client's response to the restraint device.

Reference

National Council of State Boards of Nursing. (2003). *Detailed Test Plan for the NCLEX-RN Examination.*

Chapter 7

Health Promotion and Maintenance

The Health Promotion and Maintenance category covers growth and development, disease prevention (including primary, secondary, and tertiary diseases), and lifestyle choices (including high-risk behaviors, health, and wellness). You are expected to know about families, family planning, and obstetrical and newborn care.

The test includes questions dealing with health promotion and maintenance. Remember that a great deal of nursing care is aimed toward helping patients restore health and prevent illness. Questions covering growth and development, health promotion, lifestyle choices, and how to teach patients healthy behaviors will show up here. Self-care and physical assessment are included here as well.

This is an area ripe for patient education and disease prevention. Expect questions across the lifespan requiring you to apply fundamental knowledge to complex individual, family, and community problems.

Chapter 7: Health Promotion and Maintenance

Health Promotion and Maintenance

Here are some additional topic areas and suggested study topics concerning health promotion and maintenance:

Aging process

- Nurses are expected to be familiar with changing healthcare and nursing needs across the lifespan.

- Nurses must have a working knowledge of normal and abnormal growth and development.

Ante/intra/postpartum and newborn care

- Nurses must be able to calculate an estimated date of birth and be able to participate knowledgeably in the delivery of a newborn.

- Part of the nurse's role in a maternity setting is to perform an accurate assessment of a woman who has recently delivered a child.

- Nurses are expected to know how to administer a non-stress test.

Developmental stages and transitions

- Nurses should be able to use standardized guidelines to assess a client's development.

- Based on findings about a client's development, nurses should adjust their approach to the client's care.

Health Promotion and Maintenance (cont.)

Expected body image changes

- Nurses are expected to know how to assess whether a client is adapting to physical, mental, or social changes associated with aging and other life events, e.g., pregnancy, illness.

Health and wellness

- Nurses must be able to advise clients about healthy nutritional habits that will enhance optimal weight.

- Nurses must be able to assess and interpret the client's health-related beliefs and behaviors.

Health promotion programs

- Nurses are expected to be knowledgeable and able to advise clients about health promotion activities, e.g., sun exposure, breast and testicular exams.

High-risk behaviors

- Nurses are expected to advise clients about risky behaviors and how those behaviors endanger their health, e.g., STDs, needle sharing.

Human sexuality

- Nurses are expected to be able to initiate interactions dealing with sensitive issues such as domestic abuse or sexuality.

Immunizations

- Nurses should be familiar with the Centers for Disease Control and Prevention immunization guidelines and be able to evaluate a client's immunization status.

Health Promotion and Maintenance (cont.)

Principles of teaching/learning

- Nurses must be able to evaluate the effectiveness of client teaching.

Self-care

- Nurses are expected to help clients and their families and significant others achieve self-care outcomes.

Techniques of physical assessment

- Nurses must know how to perform and what to use to complete a physical assessment.

- Nurses must understand how to asses the mental functioning of non-psychiatric clients.

Reference

National Council of State Boards of Nursing. (2003). *Detailed Test Plan for the NCLEX-RN Examination.*

Chapter 8

Psychosocial Integrity

The Psychosocial Integrity category involves therapeutic communication, psychiatric care, and family-centered care including cultural diversity issues. Other areas to expect on this portion of the test are drug abuse, end-of-life care, grief and loss, and changes in self-concept.

These questions will concern what nursing actions promote emotional and social well-being. End-of-life care has become a prominent issue in healthcare and nurses are expected to create an environment that supports death with dignity. Using therapeutic communication and creating a therapeutic environment are fundamental skills nurses must have.

What kinds of questions would you expect about psychosocial integrity? Questions in this area may well integrate a very complex illness situation with a culturally diverse family dealing with grief and loss.

Chapter 8 — Psychosocial Integrity

Psychosocial Integrity

Some suggested topic areas and examples of related content to study are:

Abuse/neglect

- Nurses must be able to identify risk factors and recognize signs of abuse that may be mental, sexual, or physical.

Behavioral interventions

- Nurses are expected to evaluate the effectiveness of any intervention by creating and using outcome objectives.

Chemical dependency

- Nurses must know how to evaluate whether the client and family are willing and able to implement the plan of care.
- Nurses must recognize when and how to change the plan.

Coping mechanisms

- Nurses must be able to evaluate how the impact of a serious and/or chronic illness is affecting the client and family's ability to provide care.

Crisis intervention

- Nurses must be able to recognize the signs of an existing or imminent crisis and be able to intervene.
- Nurse must know when and how to protect clients from self-harm.

Cultural diversity

- Nurses must understand how a client's culture will affect patient education and response to an illness.

Psychosocial Integrity (cont.)

- Nurses must understand what implications a client's culture has for the nursing care plan.

End-of-life care

- Nurses must be attentive to cultural aspects associated with death and dying and be willing to accommodate cultural concerns.

Family dynamics

- Nurses must be a guide to families in crisis.

- Nurses must recognize when parents need assistance and education about their parenting roles.

Psychopathology

- Nurses must be familiar with the signs and symptoms that accompany changes in mental status.

- Nurses are expected to recognize the manifestations of schizophrenia, bipolar disease, major depression, etc.

Religious and spiritual influences on health

- Nurses must be able to recognize and incorporate aspects of the client's spiritual and religious beliefs into the nursing plan of care.

Sensory/perceptual alterations

- Clients with altered sensory perceptions require special assessment skills that nurses must know how to perform and how to interpret, e.g., spinal cord injuries, diminished sensation in hands and feet.

Psychosocial Integrity (cont.)

Situational role changes

- Nurses must understand the importance of a client's role within his/her family, work environment, and social structure in order to provide meaningful nursing care.

Stress management

- Nurses must recognize how the stress of an illness impacts clients and family members.

Support systems

- Nurses must be able to anticipate how well a client and family will accept a plan of care and ways to adjust the plan to achieve the best compliance.

Therapeutic communications

- To be a successful practitioner, nurses must be able to recognize when communication with clients and families is effective.

Therapeutic environment

- Nurses must evaluate the client environment and make adjustments to achieve a safe and supportive environment.

Unexpected body image changes

- Nurses must recognize how a client is responding to an illness that includes changes in the client's body image.

You will be asked to apply nursing interventions to support patients' emotional and psychological needs. Don't be surprised if your answers must integrate cultural and religious beliefs as well.

Reference

National Council of State Boards of Nursing. (2003). *Detailed Test Plan for the NCLEX-RN Examination.*

Chapter 9

Physiological Integrity

Physiological integrity covers medical–surgical nursing. It includes pathophysiology, interventions, medications, and expected outcomes. You are also expected to know about diagnostic tests and laboratory values. Your understanding of pain management, including nonpharmacological measures, is also tested. Questions here will expect you to integrate what you know about disease processes with any and all possible nursing interventions.

Several subsections and sub-subsections are included in the Physiological Integrity category. The following material contains some of the general concepts included in each subsection.

Basic Care and Comfort subsection

The Basic Care and Comfort category asks you to think about less complicated, yet vitally important interventions. For example, pain is a significant issue for nurses and patients and the Joint Commission on Accreditation of Healthcare Providers pays attention to how well healthcare providers manage patients' pain. Nurses need to know interventions other than medications as ways to alleviate acute and chronic pain.

Sometimes we forget the importance of basic hygiene, movement, and sleep. The NCLEX will remind you, so think about interventions nurses use in these areas. Remember that less complicated interventions are often beneficial to patients in the intensive care unit as well as for patients in less acute settings.

Chapter 9 — Physiological Integrity

Basic Care and Comfort

Following are the key content areas included under the Basic Care and Comfort subsection of the exam, with examples of what you may be asked:

Alternative and complementary therapies

- Nurses must be familiar with various types of alternative therapies and able to explain their use to clients.

- Nurses should understand when alternative therapies are indicated.

Assistive devices

- Nurses must be able to select the appropriate device for a particular client's needs and be able to explain how to use the device correctly and safely.

- Nurses know how to use assistive devices to enhance communication and care.

Elimination

- Nurses should be able to identify factors that impact elimination.

- Nurses must be able to describe the proper procedure for inserting catheters, and for administering enemas based on client condition and therapeutic need.

Mobility/Immobility

- Nurses recognize the hazards and complications associated with immobility.

- Nurses understand good body mechanics for the nurse and client.

Basic Care and Comfort (cont.)

Nonpharmacological comfort interventions

- Nurses recognize cultural implications for pain management.

- Nurses know and initiate nonpharmacological nursing interventions for pain and injury.

- Nurses assess the client's need for pain intervention.

Nutrition and oral hydration

- Nurses must be able to apply math and statistical analysis to evaluate a client's nutrition and hydration status.

- Nurses understand the impact that disease has on nutrition and hydration.

- Nurses understand food–drug interactions and when nutritional supplements are needed.

Palliative/Comfort care

- Nurses understand the palliative care process and are able to explain and counsel clients and families about palliative care.

- Nurses know how to evaluate outcomes.

Personal hygiene

- Nurses understand the relationship between pathology and personal hygiene (e.g., oral care).

- Nurses must be able to adapt personal hygiene to patient limitations.

> ## Basic Care and Comfort (cont.)
>
> **Rest and sleep**
>
> - Nurses intervene when clients have difficulty sleeping.
>
> - Nurses must understand physiological implications of disturbed sleep patterns.

Pharmacological and Parenteral Therapies subsection

Some students may feel they need to take a pharmacology review course to prepare for NCLEX, but many choose to review pharmacology using practice NCLEX questions and questions from their pharmacology text. It's impossible for anyone to remember everything about every drug, so concentrate on classifications, such as beta blockers, and know actions, adverse reactions, drug interactions, and expected actions.

Be sure you know how to calculate a correct dosage. This section also incorporates blood administration, central lines, and other parenteral medications.

> ## Pharmacological and Parenteral Therapies
>
> Following are the key content areas included under the Pharmacological and Parenteral Therapies subsection of the exam, with examples of what you may be asked:
>
> **Adverse effects, contraindications, and side effects**
>
> - Nurses must know how to recognize and treat an allergic reaction.
>
> - Nurses know adverse reactions from drug and drug–drug interactions and are able to respond appropriately.
>
> - Nurses must be able to explain actions and potential side effects/adverse reactions to clients.

Pharmacological and Parenteral Therapies (cont.)

Blood and blood products

- Know appropriate procedures for accurate client identification to be used before administering any blood product.

- Be able to evaluate the client's response to receiving blood and blood products.

- Nurses must know the appropriate procedure for administration.

Central venous access devices

- Know the signs and symptoms of negative reactions and infections.

- Nurses must be able to provide care to clients who have a central venous access device.

Dosage calculation

- Make sure you are able to calculate the correct dose for a variety of medications.

- Know whether a dose is appropriate for the client.

Expected outcomes/effects

- Nurses must be able to determine whether the pharmacological therapeutic interventions are working as expected.

- Nurses know how to educate clients/families/significant others about prescribed medications.

Medication administration

- Understand how to dispose of medications and administration equipment appropriately.

Pharmacological and Parenteral Therapies (cont.)

- Know how to apply the five rights of medication administration.

Parenteral fluids

- Nurses calculate infusion rates and monitor the client's reactions to intravenous therapy.

- Understand the need for and procedure for administering parenteral therapy.

- Make sure you know the untoward responses.

Pharmacological interactions

- Be able to identify actual and potential drug interactions and adverse reactions.

- Be able to identify and respond to questions that require you to know if medications are pharmacologically compatible.

Pharmacological pain management

- Understand how to meet the client's need for pain management; understand how to evaluate the effectiveness of medication.

- Know the procedures for handling controlled substances.

Total parenteral nutrition (TPN)

- Nurses understand the indication for TPN.

- Nurses must be able to calculate the flow rate and monitor for adverse reactions.

- Nurses must understand how TPN is administered.

Reduction of Risk Potential subsection

In this category you will be asked to identify deviations from the normal and how to correctly gather and interpret assessment data. Don't be surprised to find assessment and laboratory data in many questions that are essentially asking about a different topic—you are expected to know how the data will guide your answer.

Reduction of Risk Potential

Following are the key content areas included under the Reduction of Risk Potential subsection of the exam, with examples of what you may be asked:

Diagnostic tests

- Understand which diagnostic tests are necessary to identify the pathophysiology that is occurring.

- Know how to perform diagnostic tests such as pulse oximeter and blood glucose, and understand what the results mean.

Laboratory values

- Be able to apply correct collection techniques.

- Nurses interpret laboratory results.

- Know values for ABGs, BUN cholesterol, glucose, hematocrit, hemoglobin, hemoglobin AiC, platelets, potassium, RBCs, sodium, urine specific gravity, and WBCs.

 Tip: These are the key lab values to focus on—you are not expected to know the value for every possible laboratory test.

Reduction of Risk Potential (cont.)

Monitoring conscious sedation

- New nurses are not expected to administer conscious sedation, however, they are expected to be able to assist and monitor the client's vital signs.

Potential for alterations in body systems

- This area includes preventing aspiration, skin breakdown, and complications of therapy and the illness.

- Be able to identify patients at risk for poor perfusion.

Potential for complications of diagnostic tests/ treatments/procedures

- Know how to perform procedures, monitor interventions, treat symptoms such as hypo/hyperglycemia, and prevent complications of treatment and disease.

- Know how to position clients for the best therapeutic effect.

- Critical-thinking skills are definitely needed here.

Potential complications from surgical procedures and health alterations

- Know how to care for pre- and post-operative patients.

- Understand the risks of surgical interventions and be able to evaluate the client's response.

Physiological Integrity — Chapter 9

Reduction of Risk Potential (cont.)

System-specific assessments

- Know the normal and abnormal assessments following surgery, a procedure, or treatment.

- Know factors that delay healing.

- Know critical values and how to apply appropriate assessment techniques.

Therapeutic procedures

- Nurses must be able to assess whether the client understands the procedure and is ready for it.

- Know how to prepare clients for procedures.

- Know how therapeutic devices work—such as chest tubes, NG tubes, and catheters—and how to care for clients that have them.

Vital signs

- Nurses must understand how to use data from vital signs to care for the client.

Physiological Adaptation subsection

The last big subsection of the test plan covers physiological integrity. As much as 70% of the test integrates questions dealing with basic care and comfort, pharmacological and parenteral therapies, reduction of risk potential, and physiological adaptation. Questions in this subsection vary from performance of basic nursing intervention to management of medical emergencies.

Watch out: This is a very comprehensive subsection and is worth spending significant time in preparation to sharpen your knowledge about the disease process and appropriate interventions. Expect to find medication calculations for such things as heparin drips and titrated homodynamic stabilizing drugs.

Physiological Adaptation

Following are the key content areas included under the Physiological Adaptation subsection of the exam, with examples of what you may be asked:

Alterations in body systems

- Questions pertaining to this section are focused on selecting appropriate nursing interventions based on the complexity and chronic nature of client illnesses.

- Be able to recognize increased intracranial pressure, know how to use complex treatments such as peritoneal dialysis, understand the implications of drainage from tubes, and so on.

Fluid and electrolyte imbalance

- Be able to recognize signs and symptoms of imbalance and know how to respond.

Hemodynamics

- Chemical reactions, cardiac function, hemodialysis, and abnormal vital signs appear here in the test plan. Again, the applicant will be expected not only to recognize the signs and symptoms, but also to apply the appropriate interventions.

Physiological Adaptation (cont.)

Illness management

- Be able to understand chronic illness and its management, along with the disease process.

Infectious disease

- Be able to recognize and provide interventions for clients with infectious diseases, including HIV-AIDS, TB, and so on.

Medical emergencies

- Be able to recognize emergency situations, and be able to respond to them. Remember the ABCs!

Radiation therapy

- Be able to recognize adverse reactions and know what can be done to minimize the negative effects of radiation.

Unexpected response to therapy

- Again, early recognition is important here.

Believe it or not, this is a smattering of the potential content area covered by NCLEX. The topics included here are intended to give you a head start with your study plan so you can identify those areas that really made you scratch your head!

Reference

National Council of State Boards of Nursing. (2003). *Detailed Test Plan for the NCLEX-RN Examination.*

Part Three

Now you know what the test covers, where do you start? This section guides you to identify the areas you need to spend most time reviewing. NCLEX success means studying smarter, not just harder, so here is all the information you need to build a study plan, boost your critical thinking, and brush up your analytical skills.

Chapter 10

Take a look at yourself— warts and all

It's study time

You're getting ready to start studying for the NCLEX and you're wondering what you need to focus on. Well, guess what? Getting ready for the NCLEX is the time to look for warts.

Fact: Now is the time to find all those undesirable shortcomings in your knowledge. You hated pediatrics and you are never going to work with children? Sorry, but questions about kids are on the NCLEX. And the computer has ways of honing in on your weakness and slamming you with question after question about—you got it—pediatrics.

That's why it is necessary to find the warts.

The National Council of State Boards of Nursing (NCSBN) says the average student spends approximately 80 hours studying for the NCLEX. If you are going to spend that much time studying for something, the logical approach is to focus on the areas that need the most work. This requires you to be brutally honest with yourself, put your pride in your pocket until after you pass, and make a list of topics in which you are weakest.

What should I do about my weak knowledge areas?

How will you know what you need to study? Use practice exam questions and think back to your nursing school experience. Did fluid and electrolytes always seem foreign? Are you glad you got through the burn unit without crashing and burning yourself? These are your areas of probable weakness.

Tip: Be brutally honest with yourself—your career is on the line.

Practice questions also help you identify your weak areas. Maybe you do well on all questions except for the ones pertaining to pharmacology. This means you should focus on drug therapy, how it works, what to expect, and so on.

Think about the tests you took throughout school. Which ones gave you the most trouble? Those are the ones to start with.

The exam before the exam

One of the best ways to identify your warts is by examining how you did in a similar test. Chances are you have already taken a big exam that will give you a pretty good understanding of your level of preparation. Many schools of nursing now require students to pass an end-of-program exam before they are eligible to apply for the NCLEX.

Though these end-of-program tests may seem like one more hurdle to overcome before you are finally finished with school, they are actually designed to prepare you for the NCLEX computer format and for the types of questions that are on the NCLEX.

If your school did require you to take one of those tests, drag out the results. Most of these tests provide detailed information to inform the student about strengths and weaknesses. Look at the feedback from those results and focus on the areas where you did poorest.

Tip: The wise graduate will look carefully and seriously at the information from the end-of-program test because the NCLEX is structured to identify your weak areas and give you lots of questions covering that material.

Think of the end-of-program test as your diagnosis, and your job is to come up with the interventions to cure the "illness." Do your results indicate that you have difficulty developing goals and a plan of care with a desirable outcome? Or do you fall short when it comes to providing integrated, cost-effective care by collaborating with members of the healthcare team? How are you at formulating hypotheses and drawing conclusions?

These seemingly abstract findings are a blueprint for your study plan.

Ask: Find out whether you will be able to "retake" a test similar to the one you took at the end of your program as practice for taking the NCLEX. This will allow you to focus on the weaknesses in your knowledge. Many times these tests are available without charge, either from your school of nursing or from the testing company in the form of a CD.

Make a list of all the areas you want to study and decide whether your knowledge is strong, basic, or weak. Spend more time on the weak areas, and less on subjects in which you are strong. A sample form is included below.

Identifying areas of weakness

Subject	My knowledge is strong	My knowledge is basic	My knowledge is weak
Endocrine	Diabetes Type II	Diabetes Type I	All other Endocrine! Especially pediatrics
Kidneys/Renal	Lab Tests	Causes of Renal disease	Difference between nephritis and nephrosis
Cardiac	Cardiac Cycle	Enzymes	Identifying Rhythms; Pediatric congenital malformations

Chapter 10   Take a look at yourself—warts and all

Study map for NCLEX preparation

This study map presents a logical process you can use to understand a client's diagnosis so that you can determine which nursing actions will enhance the client's return to optimal wellness. By working through this study map, you gain insight into how a disease process interferes with and changes the client's life. Knowing the etiology, pathophysiology, signs and symptoms, diagnostics, and medical treatments are fundamental stepping stones to planning care.

Nurses combine knowledge of diseases with the nursing process to develop and implement a plan of care. This map includes psychosocial and rehabilitation considerations to emphasize holistic nursing care and to address client needs after hospitalization.

Try using this approach to increase your understanding of any diagnoses that seem fuzzy and difficult to get your head around. Some common disease examples include: total hip arthroplasty, pancreatitis, cerebral vascular accident, renal failure, and coronary artery disease. You can insert the ones that have always given you trouble.

And don't forget you can use this approach even after you become an RN!

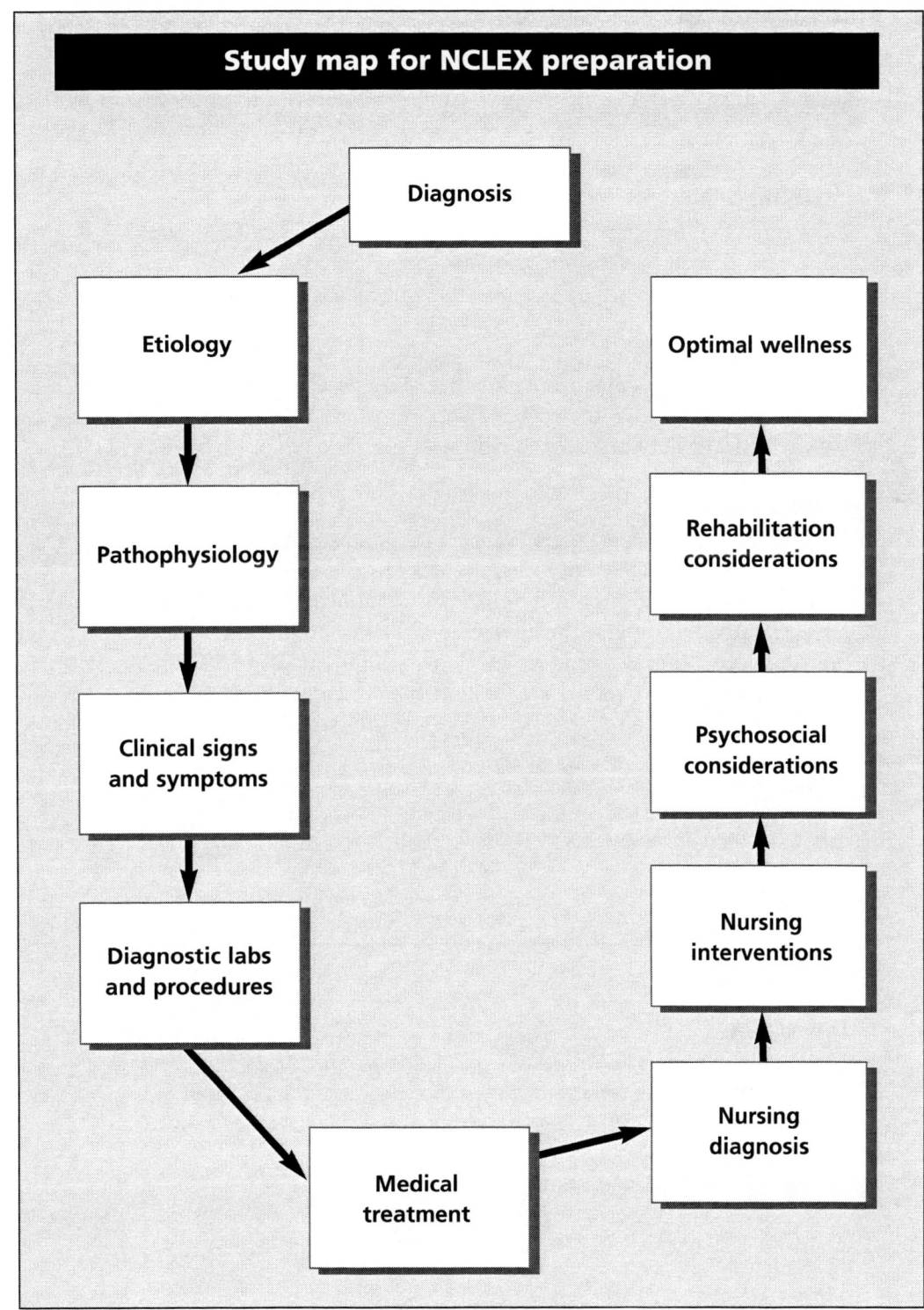

Study resources

Once you have identified your areas of weakness, you need to think about what resources can help you improve your care planning and goal development.

Textbooks
How about that nursing diagnosis book? Do you have one of the many books that describe developing good care plans? Set aside time to work through practice exercises and compare your results with the text.

Questions from your medical–surgical nursing text probably have many NCLEX-like questions that can help you analyze data to improve your ability to form hypotheses and draw conclusions. Some NCLEX resource books have sections that are designed to help with specific areas of weakness.

Review courses
A plethora of review courses are available for graduate nurses getting ready to take the NCLEX. There are courses you can take in the classroom or over the Internet, you can buy a book and study the questions, and some review books even come with supplemental CDs or online access. Almost every bookstore carries several review books with hundreds of NCLEX questions. Many study guides are reasonably priced and one of those may be all you need.

> *"I was an A student throughout nursing school, but I opted to take a review class just to feel really ready."*
>
> —C.W., recent NCLEX survivor

The NCSBN
The NCSBN offers an online review course that's available 24 hours a day. You may purchase the service for as few as four weeks for a price of $49, or for 15 weeks for $159. This may be one of the best values available.

You can get instructor feedback through discussion boards and e-mail. This may be an inexpensive option if you are self-motivated and have already identified the areas that need special focus.

Click: Visit *www.ncsbn.org* to see whether this resource is right for you.

The National League for Nursing

At the end of 2006, the National League for Nursing (NLN) launched the Simulated NCLEX-RN® Examination (SIMExam). Designed to simulate the computer-adaptive testing of the actual NCLEX, the online exam follows the eight client-need areas of the NCLEX-RN® test plan.

The simulated exam is intended to prepare students for the NCLEX and is an individualized (dependent upon each examinee's responses) test that offers a statement of performance and highlights the examinee's strengths and weaknesses in each of the content areas of the examination.

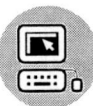

Click: Visit *www.nln.org* to find more information.

Publications

Many publishers of nursing textbooks and health-related journals offer review packages for a reasonable price that allow the student to work through a self-paced review. Other publishers offer written review packages that include CDs with test questions.

Kaplan and ATI

The Kaplan program is one of the best-known nursing review courses. Classroom, online, and home study are all available from Kaplan, which promises that anyone who is unsuccessful can repeat the course or receive their money back. Prices range from $399 for home study to $499 for classroom study. Kaplan also offers a review book with a CD that contains both questions and strategies for test taking.

ATI, a well-known national company, offers a full range of testing through schools of nursing to monitor a student's progress throughout the nursing program. These tests, along with your end-of-program exam, are good predictors of the success you'll achieve on the NCLEX. ATI also has products for NCLEX review and for sharpening critical-thinking skills. Prices are in the $350 range for a package.

Your college

Many colleges and universities offer review classes close to the time that students graduate. These courses are frequently taught by faculty and include two or more days of face-to-face classroom teaching sessions. Prices are comparable to other commercial courses and often start at $300. Check out the Web sites of the colleges near you to locate a local provider.

> *"I took a review course, but I think the most beneficial thing was reading the text and answering NCLEX-like questions. I passed!"*
>
> —L.N., brand-new RN

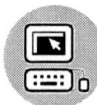

Online

Click: One nurse who wanted to help other graduates succeed on the NCLEX started a Web site that offers test-taking tips and many NCLEX-like questions. And best of all, the site is *free*. Visit Deb's NCLEX site, at *www.my-nclex-site.com*. The author has developed several clusters of test questions so that students can answer the questions, find out the correct responses, and know which areas they need to review. No matter what other resources you use, Deb's NCLEX site is definitely worth a visit.

At *www.SylviaRayfield.com*, students can sign up for a variety of learning experiences, including classroom material and self-study books with audio. Prices from this source range from $49 for books with audio to $315 for classroom study. The site claims to have a 98% to 99% passing rate among the students who have taken the courses.

Morrison Media offers a flashcard system, at *www.flashcardsecrets.com*. Click on "Vocational Exams" and find the link to NCLEX. The set contains 552 flashcards and is available for $39.95. The product comes with a one-year money-back guarantee if you don't think the flashcards are beneficial. This flashcard system uses repetition and convenience as ways to make studying for NCLEX easier.

It probably wouldn't hurt to visit a site that offers medical terminology so that you can brush up on your vocabulary. Des Moines University offers a short course on medical terminology, at *www.dmu.edu/medterms*.

New offerings appear almost weekly, so surf the Web regularly to find the review process that will work best for your style of learning. And be sure to check out *www.stressedoutnurses.com* for more tips and suggestions.

Practice makes perfect

Regardless of which review method you choose, the process of answering questions that simulate the NCLEX will help you think the way you need to think to pass the exam.

How I passed the NCLEX

> "I studied on a regular basis using books with CDs. I made myself answer 100 questions a day, read part of a study guide, and reviewed material from the last semester of classes. It paid off; I passed! But it scared me to death when the computer shut down after only 75 questions."
>
> —T.F., brand-new RN
>
> "I listened to some tapes of old lectures that I had difficulty understanding the first time I heard them. I also answered lots of questions—it felt like thousands—and I passed the test on my first try!"
>
> —M.P., brand-new RN

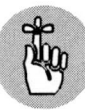

Don't forget: No matter what strategy you choose, you must be self-motivated and disciplined. The NCLEX takers who pass the first time they take the test are the ones who studied for it. Do not try to put off studying until right before you are scheduled to take the NCLEX. Think of this study time as short-term pain for long-term gain.

References

National League for Nursing. (2006). "Executive Report." Special issue of *Shaping the Future.* Fall 2006 (11).

Chapter 11

Develop a study plan

What don't you know?

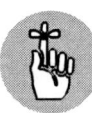

Don't forget: Regardless of the number of questions you have to answer on the NCLEX, you have only about a minute to spend on each question. The test is designed to quickly identify your weakest areas and to give you questions in those areas. Each subsequent question will be more difficult than the preceding one. Consequently, if you focus your studying efforts on the areas in which you are strong, you may fail the NCLEX because of the way the computer will select questions for you.

Watch out: The bottom line is that you must identify your weaknesses and focus on those areas when you study for the NCLEX.

Tips for successful studying: Have a plan

Want an easy way to pass the NCLEX? The answer is simple. Start studying early. The NCLEX is not a test you can cram for the night before.

If you are at the end of your nursing program, this tip won't help you much, but if you are still immersed in nursing school, now is the time to get into the habit of studying regularly.

Chapter 11 — Develop a study plan

Tip: What you learn in nursing school is cumulative and you continue to build on it throughout your career. Instead of cramming right before each test, establish a regular study schedule. Most of the time what you stuff into your brain when you cram you end up forgetting as rapidly as you learned it.

Try a different method. Review class notes the night after the class and make sure you read the textbook. Most programs provide you with objectives and content outlines for each course. Get into the habit of answering the objectives and finding the content in the text that corresponds with the content outline. You will not only get a jump on coursework and the NCLEX, but also be a much better nurse.

Start with a study plan

The first order of business is to develop a study plan. Even before graduation, explore study options and decide whether you will take a review course.

Tip: Registering early for review courses sometimes gets you a nice discount.

Once you have decided whether you will take a review course, you can determine your study schedule. Some students think a schedule is not necessary, but most who were successful on the NCLEX stuck to a pretty rigid study schedule. Get yourself a calendar and specify the times and days you will be studying. Mark them off as though they are the most important appointments you have ever had—they may be!

Let your friends and family know that your study time is sacred and that you cannot be disturbed!

Don't procrastinate

Start studying early. Don't wait until the week before you are scheduled to take the NCLEX to begin studying for it. Lay out a schedule with specific topics, and targets of what you want to accomplish knowledge-wise about the topics. For example, do you need to have a better understanding of the intra-partum period, or are those growth and development milestones still not part of your fundamental knowledge base? Lay out a plan to correct your deficits.

Here is a sample study plan to get you thinking. You can create your own and fill in the topic areas you want to study.

Study plan

Subject/topic to be studied	Date	✓
Review A and P Cardiac: know flow of drop of blood, electrical impulse transmission, S1 and S2, major coronary arteries	Start 1/3/07 for 3 days; 2 hours a day	
Review growth and development across the lifespan; including normal physiological changes with aging	Start 1/3/07 for 2 days; 1 hour a day	
Review A and P along with pathophysiology of endocrine system. Study origins of hormones and target organs. Know effects of hypo and hyper secretion. Know treatment and nursing interventions	Start 1/06/07 for 4 days 3 hours a day	

Find your zone
Test-savvy experts recommend that you designate your study place. Dedicate a particular spot that you will devote solely to studying for the NCLEX. Consider your telephone or cell phone off-limits in this area. You may need to inform your family/roommates that you are not to be disturbed when you are in "study heaven."

Consider posting a "do not disturb" sign on your door when you are studying to ensure you get the peace and quiet you need. See the end of this chapter for a sign you can use.

Stick to a routine
Create a routine and stick to it. If you are best early in the morning, dedicate that time to studying. Set aside one or two hours, three, four, or more days a week, to studying for the NCLEX—allow nothing to interfere. As part of your study plan, rotate topics to prevent boredom and disinterest.

Prioritize
Arrange your work schedule to complement your study time. Do not feel pressured into taking extra shifts that cut into your study schedule. Remember, you are getting ready to change jobs.

Concentrate
Focus! All of us find our mind wanders when we are engaged in a "must do" activity. Pay attention to when your mind is wandering and gently bring yourself back to the here and now. You might even repeat a phrase to yourself when you catch yourself wandering. Something such as "I am an RN" might get your attention back on task.

Change it up
Put some variety into your study plan. Reading is important, but it may become tedious after a while. So, interject some homemade or professional flashcards, NCLEX questions, a trip to the Web for images, or a study session with a friend who is on the same wavelength to break up the monotony. Many experts advocate making learning an active process, so create games to help retain your learning. And remember, you can't possibly answer too many practice questions.

Friends with benefits
If you want to study with friends, many people find study groups very helpful and successful. You determine what works for you. If you have always

studied alone and have done well, the NCLEX is probably not the time to make a drastic change in your habits. With that said, sometimes sharing thoughts and ideas with friends who are also studying can be a great asset. Choose wisely and don't make study groups your only study method.

> "I studied with the same friends I studied with during school. We knew each other's weaknesses and forced each other to work on those areas. It really helped and we all passed!"
>
> —L.F., brand-new RN

Treat yourself

Yes, you are entitled to breaks and some rewards. Get up, walk around, stretch, or eat something you love (the NCLEX study period is probably not the best time to start a new diet). Stay hydrated and avoid overdoing the caffeine. Reward yourself! Get that hot chocolate with whipped cream at your favorite coffee shop. Be your best friend—the two of you are in this together.

Top 10 study tips that work

1. Develop a study plan.
2. Give yourself enough time to study.
3. Create a "study place" that is free of distractions.
4. Develop goals for your study periods.
5. Focus and bring your wandering mind back to the task at hand.
6. Develop a routine and establish a time to study.
7. Study when you are at your peak.
8. Vary your study activities; don't bore yourself.
9. Use what you know about your weaknesses to help focus your study plan.
10. Reward yourself—you deserve it!

Develop a study plan — Chapter 11

Do not disturb studying sign

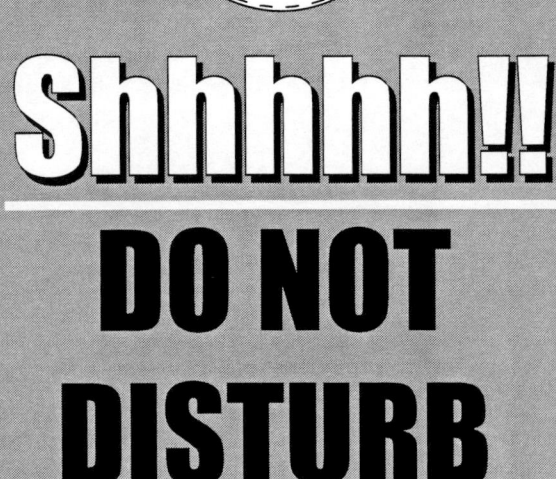

Chapter 12

Critical thinking and the NCLEX

Critical thinking: The pathway to success

In nursing school, how many times did your theory and clinical instructor tell you to use your critical-thinking skills? Now those skills are going to come in handy. The NCLEX is the culmination of every situation that required your critical-thinking skills.

What is critical thinking?

You know everyone talks about critical thinking, but you may be confused about what it actually means. Well, the good news is that critical thinking is so fundamental to nursing practice that nurses do it automatically.

Critical thinking can be defined as an organized, cognitive process; a way of identifying underlying assumptions in a situation; and a method for exploring alternatives and selecting the best approach to a situation.

Chapter 12: Critical thinking and the NCLEX

Am I a critical thinker?

Characteristics of critical thinkers

- Open-minded
- Asks questions
- Displays curiosity
- Reasons
- Thinks independently
- Analytical
- Explores consequences
- Awareness of strengths and weaknesses
- Ability to see things from more than one perspective
- Ongoing striving for improvement

Strategies used in critical thinking

- Reasoning
- Pattern recognition
- Repetitive hypothesizing
- Mental representation
- Intuition

Source: Critical Thinking in the Emergency Department: Skills to Assess, Analyze, and Act. *(2006) Shelley Cohen, RN, BS, CEN. Marblehead, MA: HCPro, Inc.*

Critical thinking and the NCLEX — Chapter 12

Do I have critical-thinking skills?

Remember when you were gathering information to prepare for a clinical day and you had to put the pieces together so you would know how to approach your patient? Well, taking the NCLEX requires the same process. All of those clinical preps you have done will help you with NCLEX—aren't you glad that hard work will finally pay off?

Using critical thinking in the NCLEX

The key to using critical-thinking skills is to remain open to possibilities. For example, thinking critically involves identifying the variables in the situation, analyzing how each variable fits and interacts with the other variables, deciding which variable(s) is (are) most important, and finally assessing the correctness of your thinking process.

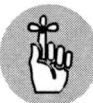

Don't forget: The starting point for this critical-thinking process during NCLEX is to figure out what the question is asking.

You may be asking yourself two questions:

1. What can I do between now and the time I take the NCLEX to sharpen my critical-thinking skills?

2. How do I apply critical-thinking skills when I am taking the NCLEX exam?

The long and short answer is that you PRACTICE! Get your hands on as many NCLEX-like questions as you can. Do not simply whiz through them as fast as possible. Instead, make sure you understand what the question is asking. Take time to analyze how you came to the answer you chose.

Here are two techniques you can use to boost your critical-thinking skills and to aid you during the test.

Think about the nursing process

Don't forget that critical thinking and the nursing process go hand in hand. If you feel at a loss when facing a question, then fall back on that old friend: nursing process. The nursing process is a roadmap for critical thinking and it will provide a starting point when you feel lost.

First read the question and ask yourself, "Where in the nursing process am I?" Once you recognize whether the question is about assessing, diagnosing, planning, intervening, or evaluating, then you will be able to use critical thinking to identify the answer choices that match the appropriate part of the nursing process. A question that asks you about nursing interventions means you have to look for the response that includes an action the nurse must take.

Give the technique a try when you are studying with practice questions:

1. Read the question.

2. Ask yourself to which part of the nursing process the question applies.

Think about the variables

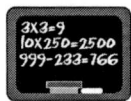

Example: Let's say you are presented with a question concerning delegation of nursing duties to a licensed practical nurse (LPN) or nursing assistant. Typically a question like this will give you four patient situations and ask you which patient you would delegate to the LPN.

1. The first step in critical thinking is to identify the variables in the situation, i.e., how stable is each patient and is the task to be delegated within the scope of practice for the LPN?

2. The next step is to consider how the task and the stability of the patient interact.

    - Is the patient stable and the task beyond the scope of practice because it involves assessing the patient?

    - Is the task within the scope of an LPN's practice but the patient is unstable enough to require an RN's care?

3. The final step is to ask yourself if you are comfortable with your thinking process.

Believe it or not, this critical-thinking process is done in seconds and you will have time to go through this process during the test.

Tip: Of course, you will be better at this process if you have practiced ahead of time. That's why doing practice questions is so useful.

Critical thinking and the NCLEX — Chapter 12

"I was unsuccessful on my first try, so I'm forcing myself to do at least 50 practice questions each day to sharpen my critical-thinking skills."

—K.V., about to retake the NCLEX

"I studied like a maniac. During NCLEX all I could think of was 'use critical thinking, use critical thinking.' I know those practice questions paid off."

—F.C., recently successful at NCLEX

"All during the test I kept saying to myself, am I using my critical-thinking skills? I think they have become second nature now."

—L.C., recently passed on first try

Chapter 13

Test-taking strategies

Taking tests is not new to you. You have likely already developed some strategies that work and at the same time, you probably have some habits that interfere with your best test-taking efforts. This chapter offers some suggestions for maximizing your success. You'll find some hints about using study time well and you'll learn some tactics for taking the question apart to help you select the best answer.

Reading the question

Watch out: It doesn't get more fundamental than this. You are probably asking yourself, how can I possibly answer the question without reading it first? But think about it. Have you ever missed a question because the stem said something like, "Which of the following actions is not likely to cause post-operative bleeding" and your eyes missed the 'not?' Often, our eyes will skip right over that crucial word. We will be looking for a cause for post-operative bleeding and miss the actual point of the question. Reading the question to clearly understand what it asks is a basic technique that can be sharpened with practice.

Here's a sample question from the NCLEX free test prep review site, *www.nclexinfo.com*.

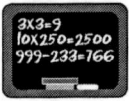

Example: A patient has a history of ketoacidosis. Which of the following would you not expect to see with this patient if this condition were acute?

Take the question apart. See that NOT in there? You are looking for the answer that is not associated with ketoacidosis. Think about what you know about ketoacidosis. It occurs in individuals with Type I diabetes mellitus, right? Those individuals exhibit the "polys"—polyuria, polydipsia, polyphagia. They eat, drink, and urinate a lot.

So the answer choices are:

a. vomiting
b. extreme thirst
c. weight gain
d. acetone breath smell

Let's critically think through the answers. Vomiting may be related to the underlying disease that brought on the ketoacidosis. Extreme thirst is polydipsia, one of the expected symptoms. Acetone breath smell is that fruity smell so characteristic of patients in ketoacidosis. But patients with Type I diabetes are notoriously thin because their bodies cannot use the food they ingest. They have no insulin and that is why they eat (polyphagia) all the time. Therefore the logical answer is "c" weight gain, as you would not expect this with this patient.

Here's another one.

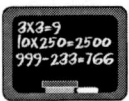

Example: The physician inserts a central catheter to administer parenteral nutrition. The solution is to be started as soon as x-ray confirms the placement of the catheter. The x-ray shows the tip of the catheter in the superior vena cava. The appropriate action for the nurse is to

a. start the solution at the prescribed rate
b. notify the physician that the catheter needs adjustment
c. wait for further orders from the physician
d. insert the catheter by an additional 3cm so it is positioned correctly

Choice d can be eliminated immediately—nurses do not insert central catheters. Choice c puts the nurse in the position of doing nothing for a patient ill enough to need parenteral nutrition. How long would you wait? This is not a viable choice. To answer this question correctly, the nurse should think about where the tip of the catheter is supposed to be.

The superior vena cava is the correct place for the catheter to be. Any farther and it would enter the atria and interfere with cardiac function. Therefore the correct answer is a.

Understanding the question

Another issue associated with reading the question concerns language arts. Two skills are involved here. One skill involves your vocabulary. Have you been struggling to understand your textbooks and lectures because there were so many words you did not understand? The second skill has to do with your ability to decipher what an unfamiliar word means by examining the context or by breaking the word apart into syllables that tell you what the word means.

Many schools of nursing require entering students to take tests that measure the student's reading ability. Go back to the results of those tests and determine if your reading level needs a boost. If so, take a look at some of the resources your school offers to help you with comprehension and vocabulary. Start there first. Remember, the nursing school has a vested interest in helping you be successful on NCLEX.

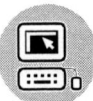

Click: You can also find resources on the Web. Google the topic and you will find some ideas for improving your reading comprehension.

Practice

Tip: Make yourself practice using the correct verbiage to describe your nursing findings and avoid using the jargon of the day even if your friends think you sound weird. Vocabulary flashcards may be helpful to familiarize yourself with new words.

Consider reviewing medical terminology, including the prefixes and suffixes that facilitate interpretation of the root word. You can find helpful terminology books at the library or in a bookstore.

Click: Two helpful Web sites for improving your vocabulary are *Medical Terminology* (*http://ec.hku.hk/mt/*) and Des Moines University's Short Course in Medical Terminology (*www.dmu.edu/medterms*). Both provide medical terminology, including in-depth discussion of prefixes, suffixes, and root words. They also offer useful links for anatomy reviews. These are free sites, so take advantage of them if you have any questions about whether your vocabulary skills are up to speed.

The Des Moines University site offers a course and has terminology broken down by body system. Nursing students who have used it rave about how much it has helped them. Getting the lingo down speeds up your ability to read and comprehend questions on the NCLEX.

> *Brushing up on terminology can make a big difference in your comprehension. L.L. is a first semester nursing student who tried the Des Moines University site and improved his terminology: "Suddenly it began to make sense. I don't struggle with every word and need a dictionary just to read an assignment."*
>
> —L.L.

The NCLEX review site *www.nclexinfo.com* also has information on study guides and a flashcard review to help with medical terminology.

English as a second language

If your first language is not English, you may face special vocabulary and grammar challenges. Think about how well you did on tests in nursing school and whether an English refresher course would be useful to you. A class may help increase your understanding of the nuances of English.

Check out the colleges in your area—they may have special funds to assist students with language skills.

> *"As a native of Hong Kong, English is not my first language. So throughout nursing school I worked to increase my vocabulary and understanding of English. I was successful the first time I took the NCLEX."*
>
> —W.V., recent graduate

Chapter 14

Choosing the right answer

How do I decide between two right answers?

The questions on the NCLEX present you with many varied patient and practice situations. Count on every multiple choice question that asks you to select the ONE best choice to have at least two plausible answers. Your job is to choose the one best answer.

Here are three techniques teachers advocate when practicing:

1. Cover the answers with your hand, read the question, and try to answer it without uncovering the answers. Then look for the answer that is closest to your response.
2. Read the question and try each answer. Ask yourself whether the answer is true and settle on the one that is most true.
3. Cover the question and just look at the answers. From the answers, try to figure out what the question would be for each answer (like contestants do on the quiz show Jeopardy!) Compare each question you come up with to the actual question. The answer that answers both your made up question and the one on the test is probably the correct answer to the test question.

Chapter 14 **Choosing the right answer**

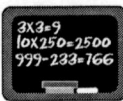

Example: Here's a question dealing with preparing a patient for a diagnostic procedure. This question asks the nurse to arrange the patient in the best possible position for a thoracentesis.

First, you must know that a thoracentesis is a procedure that requires inserting a tube into the chest cavity to withdraw fluid, or inserting a chest tube. The nurse must position the patient so that there is room between the ribs to access the intercostals space, so the tube can enter the thoracic cavity.

If the question gives you the following choices, ask yourself which of these positions will open the space between the ribs and expose the intercostals space:

   a. lying supine

   b. lying prone

   c. in the sitting position

   d. in semi-Fowler's position

That's right; the best position to choose is the sitting position. Usually in this position, the patient will be leaning forward with his or her arms elevated. The other positions do not expose the intercostals space nearly as well.

I'm still unsure

If you have tried these techniques and you are still baffled, try rereading the question. Look carefully for words or phrases that provide a clue you missed the first time. Look for qualifiers such as *always, never, none,* and *all*—it is unlikely that those words are in the correct choice. After you have made up your mind, stick with your first hunch. Don't change your answer unless you thought of new information that clearly changes your choice.

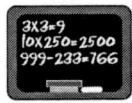

Example: Here's a question you could answer using this technique.

Which of the following statements is true of health and illness?

   a. Health and illness are the same for all people.

   b. Health and illness are individually defined by each person.

   c. People with chronic illnesses are never healthy.

   d. People with chronic illnesses have poor health beliefs.

You can eliminate choice "a" right off the bat because of the "all" statement. Similarly, you can eliminate choice "c" because of the word never. You should eliminate choice "d" because it makes a value judgment about people with chronic illnesses as a group. The only choice left is "b." Read the answer and see whether it makes sense to you. Yes, it does. So, that is the answer.

Should I guess?

The NCLEX format requires that you select your answer and confirm it before moving on. The next question will not appear until you confirm your answer. Consequently, you are required to guess if you don't know the answer; which means you must unleash your critical thinking skills and select the answer that makes the most sense to you. Use the processes just described to analyze the question and eliminate wrong answers so that you can choose the best remaining response. Remember, you probably know more than you think.

Tip: Stay calm when time is getting short, and do not use "rapid guessing" to answer any remaining questions. Most experts agree that rapid guessing can drastically lower a test score. It is better to run out of time.

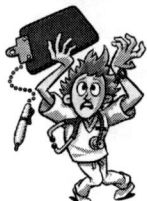

Don't panic: Your preparation with hundreds of test questions and vocabulary enhancers, along with those critical-thinking skills, are your best hedge when you have to guess or decide between two answers that "are right." Being well prepared gives you confidence that you will be able to analyze each question and identify the best answer.

Question dissection

Let's consider some other tactics you can use to quickly pull a question apart. Start by reading the question carefully. Be sure you understand what the question is asking. Look for qualifiers such as *all, none, every, except,* and so on. If the question still seems mystifying, look for any part that is familiar—a laboratory value or nursing diagnosis—to provide some guidance for your selection. Is this question similar to a previous one, and can you use that information for some help?

If two answers seem the same, look for the one that is more inclusive. Watch out for questions and answers with negatives that cancel each other. Options that are completely unfamiliar to you are probably not correct. Similarly, answers that don't fit grammatically with the question are probably not correct either. Some questions may have parallel answer choices, with one serving as a decoy (e.g., "raises the blood pressure" and "lowers the blood pressure"). One of those is probably the correct choice.

Sometimes it helps to give each answer the "true/false" test. Read each answer and ask yourself whether it is true or false as a way to help narrow down multiple choices. Remember, you are not just looking for the correct answer. You must identify the "best" answer in order to get the question right.

Last but not least, be sure to read all directions carefully; be sure you know what the question is asking you to do. And pace yourself; you have approximately one minute for each question. One minute is longer than you think.

Tip: As part of your test preparation, set a timer when you run through practice questions. Soon you will develop an inner sense of how long a minute feels, which will help you on the actual day.

Quick tips to break down the question

- Read the question
- Understand what the question is asking
- Look for qualifiers such as all, none, every, except
- Look for something familiar
- Give each answer the true/false test
- If you still don't know, make an educated guess

Chapter 15

Topics for serious review

Basic areas for serious review

The NCLEX was created based on Bloom's taxonomy of cognitive domain learning. Remember, we discussed Bloom in a previous chapter. The lower levels of Bloom are not used. According to his taxonomy, knowledge questions that simply require memorization are the lowest-level and easiest questions to answer.

The NCLEX focuses on application of complex thought processes to resolve complex patient situations. Knowledge of basic facts such as routine laboratory values is assumed. The test requires that you understand what implications for nursing care are inherent in a patient's laboratory results. You will be required to analyze and synthesize information to solve patient care situations.

The NCLEX is based on a test plan that designates percentages for each area of the plan. Every candidate receives questions consistent with the test plan. The two main areas of testing are client needs and integrated processes. The client needs area is further broken down into four main categories that are subdivided into six subsections, as shown in the following box. You can find additional detailed information in Part II.

Chapter 15: Topics for serious review

NCLEX–RN® client areas

Safe and Effective Care Environment
    Management of Care
    Safety and Infection Control
Health Promotion and Maintenance
Psychosocial Integrity
Physiological Integrity
    Basic Care and Comfort
    Pharmacological and Parenteral Therapies
    Reduction of Risk Potential
    Physiological Adaptation

Integrated processes within the test plan include nursing processes; caring; communication and documentation; and teaching and learning. These areas are part of each question, and they can guide your interpretation of each question. Ask yourself, "Is this question about the nursing process, caring, communication, or teaching," as a way to help you identify the type of answer you are looking for.

Part II describes test plan components further. There is no way to know how many questions from any one category you will receive on the test; however, the current proportions from each category are consistent from test to test.

The test is designed to make candidates think about nursing actions. Knowing when you are capable of handling the situation and when to call a physician is an important critical-thinking skill. Patient safety and prevention of complications are part of this cognitive process. Seek out practice questions that require you to determine appropriate nursing actions in a variety of patient care scenarios.

Select practice questions that challenge you to stretch your knowledge. At first, you may need to start with less complex items. But really push yourself so that you will be functioning at a cognitive level that is consistent with test expectations. Don't get discouraged if you have difficulty answering hard questions; just keep plugging away until you fine-tune your analytical skills. Remember, you can dissect each question to figure out the answer. During practice sessions, make question dissection a tool that sharpens your critical-thinking skills.

Laboratory values

It is important to know the following laboratory values when taking the NCLEX:

- Arterial Blood Gases (ABGs): Know the normal values for pH, PO_2, PCO_2, SaO_2, HCO

- Blood Urea Nitrogen (BUN): What it measures, what do increases indicate, what nursing interventions are used?

- Cholesterol (total): Why is cholesterol important, what pathophysiology is related to elevated cholesterol, what medications would you expect the patient to receive?

- Glucose: What are the therapeutic ranges, how are hypoglycemia and hyperglycemia treated, what signs and symptoms would the patient be exhibiting?

- Hematocrit: What is the significance of hematocrit, what conditions cause elevations or below normal values, how is hematocrit related to hydration?

- Hemoglobin: What are the normal ranges for men and women, why would the hemoglobin be elevated or too low, what treatments would you expect the patient with high or low hemoglobin to receive, what are the signs and symptoms of high and low hemoglobin?

- Hemoglobin AiC: How is this laboratory value used in the care of patients with diabetes, what is the desirable level?

- Platelets: What do platelets do, what drugs effect them, what is the normal range?

- Potassium (K): What is the therapeutic range for potassium, what is its chemical sign, what are the signs of hypokalemia and hyperkalemia?

- Red Blood Cells (RBC): What are the normal values for men and women, what does erythropoietin do for red blood production, what are the signs and symptoms of elevated and low RBCs?

- Sodium (Na): What is the primary action of sodium in the body, how does it help regulate hydration, what are the signs and symptoms of hypernatremia and hyponatremia?

- Urine: What is the normal range of specific gravity, why is specific gravity important?

- White Blood Cells (WBC): What is the normal range for white blood cells, what does a shift to the left mean, what are the different WBCs and what does each type do in the body?

A question about laboratory values may appear this way:

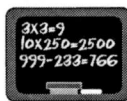

Example: As the nurse is preparing to draw blood for a hematocrit, the patient asks what the test is for. The best response from the nurse is:

a. It measures the oxygen-carrying capacity of blood.

b. It lets us determine how many red blood cells you have.

c. It tells us how effectively you use oxygen.

d. It gives us the percentage by volume of red blood cells in your blood.

The question is not asking you the normal value of a hematocrit. You need to understand what information is learned from the hematocrit. What is your choice for the answer?

A hematocrit simply tells you the percentage of red blood cells—it doesn't tell you about the use of oxygen, how many red blood cells you have, or how much oxygen is carried. Think about the lab results you have seen to help you discriminate among the answers.

Don't be surprised if "call the physician" appears as a choice in several questions. The key things to focus on for these questions is "Do I have the information I need to explain the situation to the physician, or do I need to perform further assessments before I call the physician?" Many times you need to gather more information before calling the doctor.

Making safe choices
The NCLEX is about determining whether you have enough knowledge to practice as a minimally competent practitioner. If you find choices to

questions that advocate unsafe nursing practice, you can eliminate those choices. Unsafe practice is never an option.

When you have narrowed down your choices to the two that seem right, you should ask yourself whether one of the responses is safer than the other. The safest response is the better choice.

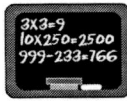

Example: Which of the following medications would be administered to a patient who had an MI within the last four hours?

    a. streptokinase

    b. atropine sulfate

    c. acetaminophen

    d. warfarin (Coumadin)

To answer this, you must know the safe parameters for administration of streptokinase, which is the correct answer because the patient is within the allowable time frame for the drug to be used to break up the clot.

Earlier, we emphasized the importance of reading the question correctly. An important part of reading the question is being sure you understand what the words mean. Don't mistake similar-looking or similar-sounding words. It can make a 100% difference in terms of whether you get the right answer.

For example, the following question from the NCLEX test site contains sound-alike terms:

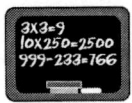

Example: A nurse is administering a shot of vitamin K to a 30-day-old infant. Which of the following target areas is the most appropriate?

    a. gluteus maximus

    b. gluteus minimus

    c. vastus lateralis

    d. vastus medialis

This question involves sound-alike words and the candidate must discriminate among these choices. Further, the candidate needs to think about giving an infant an injection and the implications of that. The best choice here is vastus lateralis.

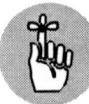

Don't forget: Bone up on your vocabulary to make sure you understand what is being asked. This is easy with the Web resources available, and it will definitely pay off.

So far, you have explored how to apply for the NCLEX, what the test is like, how your score is calculated, and some methods to approach test questions that will help you choose the correct answer. The next section gives you some hints about how to take care of yourself so that you will be in the best possible frame of mind for taking the NCLEX.

Chapter 16

If they passed, so can you

I think I'm going to fail

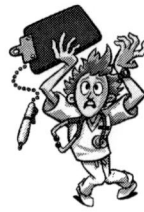

Don't panic: There is no question that the NCLEX is a stressful time, but don't stress yourself out too much. The success rate for passing the NCLEX is high. Keep in mind that your school of nursing designed a curriculum that provided the information you need to pass the NCLEX and be a safe beginning practitioner. Your nursing school is vested in you passing the NCLEX. You have already been taught everything you will need to know to pass.

If more than a million people have passed, so can I

Fact: Take comfort in the numbers. The National Council of State Boards of Nursing (NCSBN) publishes the pass rates for the NCLEX. More than one million people (1,253,972) have passed the NCLEX-RN in the past 10 years. That's 71.88%—or 7 out of 10 people—of everyone who took the test (NCSBN 2006).

These numbers were for total NCLEX-RN takers, but it gets even better if you were educated in the United States and you are taking the test for the first time. In the last 10 years, 85.8% of U.S. educated, first-time takers have passed the NCLEX-RN (NCSBN 2006).

Chapter 16 — If they passed, so can you

Pass rate breakdown

In the first nine months of 2006 (the latest figures available at publication), 76.7% of NCLEX-RN candidates passed. See the table below for a breakdown.

2006 NCLEX-RN® volume and pass rate

Candidates	# testing	% passing
First-time	119,579	84.9
Repeat	28,726	42.5
U.S. educated	117,538	84.1
Internationally educated	30,767	48.4
RN total	**148,305**	**76.7**

Source: National Council of State Boards of Nursing

The pass rates for diploma, ADN, BSN, and foreign graduates from January through December 2005 appear in the following table.

If they passed, so can you — Chapter 16

2005 NCLEX-RN® pass rate breakdown

First time, U.S. educated	# testing	% passing
RN–Diploma	3,540	90.3
RN–ADN	60,053	87.5
RN–BSN	35,496	86.7
TOTAL First time, U.S. educated	**99,187**	**87.3**
Repeat, U.S. educated	21,964	53.6%
First time, internationally educated	17,980	58.1
Repeat, internationally educated	15,765	27.3%
ALL CANDIDATES	**154,896**	**73.0%**

Source: National Council of State Boards of Nursing

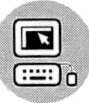

Click: You can find pass results for your state. Just search on your state's Board of Nursing Web site.

As you can see, the pass rates are relatively high, indicating congruence between RN nursing school curriculum and passing the NCLEX. You may notice that foreign-educated nurses often have more difficulty with the NCLEX. There are indications that language is the greatest barrier for foreign graduates to overcome. English is a difficult language and has some interesting nuances, such as different words pronounced the same way (e.g., red and read). Other speculation is that the curriculum and clinical experience in other countries are different from those in the United States.

Students graduating from U.S. schools of nursing have an excellent chance of passing the NCLEX. Also, first-time takers do better than repeaters, so you will want to pull out all the stops to get yourself ready for the NCLEX. In addition, studies indicate that the sooner you take the test after graduation, the better your chances are for passing. So, get your studying done and your application filed as quickly as you can.

> *"I needed to take a couple of courses after the nursing program before I was eligible to take the NCLEX and it really hurt my NCLEX preparation and I had to repeat. I recommend taking the NCLEX as quickly as possible after you finish your nursing program."*
>
> —T.Y., now a successful RN
>
> *"I got my application in as soon as I could and still had to wait over a month to get an available date because so many people were taking the test at that time. It worried me—but I passed!"*
>
> —M.J., recent NCLEX taker
>
> *"I ended up traveling to another city so I could take the test as soon as possible. I didn't want to start a new job and try to get ready for NCLEX at the same time."*
>
> —M.P., recent NCLEX taker

References

NCSBN. 2006. Accessed from *www.ncsbn.org* on December 1, 2006.

Part Four

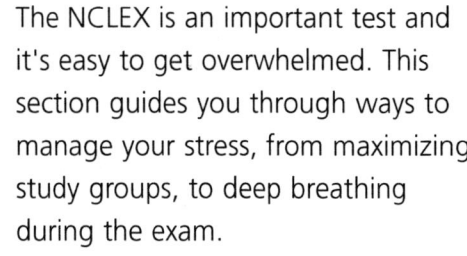

The NCLEX is an important test and it's easy to get overwhelmed. This section guides you through ways to manage your stress, from maximizing study groups, to deep breathing during the exam.

Chapter 17

Take a deep breath

Is it any wonder that you feel stressed? You've been working toward becoming a nurse for so long. And now, just one test stands between you and your goal.

If you have a lot of stress in your life already, the looming NCLEX is only going to add more stress. This means you risk becoming overwhelmed and making everything more difficult than it ought to be. Getting a handle on your stress is the first problem you should tackle.

How stressful is your life?

Stress is the number-one health problem in America, and job stress is the major culprit. Nursing can be a stressful profession, especially depending on where you work and how you handle stress in your daily life.

Watch out: People become stressed and burned out because they think they have little control over their environment and their future. Do not fall into this trap. *Focus on what you can control* and you will realize that there are many things you can do to improve your environment.

Chapter 17 Take a deep breath

How stressful is your life? (cont.)

When you learn how to manage your stress, you can experience life from a more positive perspective. In fact, studies have shown that when we view stress as a positive rather than a negative experience, it leads us to happier and more fulfilled lives.

Before we delve into skills for handling stress, take the test shown in the following figure to determine the level of stress you are currently facing. To calculate your total stress points, add up those life events you have experienced in the past year.

See the next page for a sample life event stress test.

If your total score for this activity is less than 150 points, you have a low susceptibility to developing a stress-related illness. If, however, you scored more than 150 points, you have a 50% chance of developing a stress-related illness in the near future. If you scored more than 300 points, you have a 90% chance of developing a stress-related illness in the near future. Anyone with a score of 150 or more should learn and practice stress management.

Source: Patricia Duclos-Miller, MS, RN, CNA, BC. 2006. Stressed Out About Your First Year of Nursing. Marblehead, MA: HCPro, Inc.

Life event stress test

Life event	Points	Life event	Points	Life event	Points
Death of a spouse or partner	100	Significant change to financial status	37	Trouble with employer	23
Divorce	73	Death of a close friend	36	Change in working hours or conditions	20
Marital separation	65	Change in line of work	35	Moving house	20
Serving a jail sentence	63	Increase in domestic arguments	35	Changing school	20
Death of a close relative	63	Large mortgage	31	Change in recreation	20
Serious illness or injury	53	Foreclosure of mortgage or loan	30	Change in church activities	19
Marriage	50	More or less responsibility at work	29	Change in social life	19
Loss of job	47	Child leaving home	29	Taking out a small mortgage	17
Marital reconciliation	45	Friction with in-laws	29	Sleep problems	16
Retirement	45	Outstanding personal achievement	28	Change in family get-togethers	15
Change in family member's health	44	Spouse starting or ending work	26	Change in eating habits	15
Pregnancy	40	Starting or completing education	26	Going on vacation	13
Sexual difficulties	39	Change in living conditions	25	Christmas	12
New baby or family member	39	Change in personal habits	24	Minor violation of the law	11

Your overall score: _____

Source: Gill, Jit. 2003. Stress Survival Guide. NY: HarperTorch.

How stressed are you?

The good news is that stress in manageable amounts is actually a good thing. It speeds up the heart rate and sends blood to the brain. Remember, stress accelerates the sympathetic nervous system. Our goal now is to figure out how to keep enough stress in our lives to stay sharp without succumbing to its negative effects.

Ask: Let's take an NCLEX stress test.

Are you stressed?

Answer the following questions:

- Are your shoulders too close to your earlobes?
- Are you tapping or shaking your foot or finger?
- Do you feel tired enough that you could lie down and take a nap?
- Are you worrying about what happened yesterday or the day before?
- Do you think everyone will be successful but you?
- Are you feeling on edge?
- Is your breathing shallow?

If you answered yes to any of these questions, you are overstressed. As a nurse, you know how dangerous too much stress can be. Your blood pressure goes up, often to unhealthy levels; you put out excess adrenaline that is stimulating at first, but over time makes it difficult to focus and concentrate.

Stress, called "tension of the mind" in some cultures, can be redirected. First, we have to acknowledge the stress, and second, we must make a conscious effort to dispel it. So, let's explore some methods for reducing that unnecessary stress.

Free, easy, and available now

Fact: First things first: There's a quick, easy, and, most important, free way to relieve your stress that you can try right now and feel better instantly.

Smile!

Smiling doesn't cost anything and can be a great stress buster. Think about when you see someone walking around with a big frown on his or her face. What does this tell you? Do you think that person is happy, sad, relaxed, or stressed?

That's right, you immediately think he or she is unhappy and stressed. Researchers have demonstrated the connection between production of neurotransmitters and hormones and the stress we feel. The simple act of smiling reduces production of those neurotransmitters and hormones and, thus, changes our physiology.

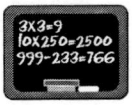

Example: Try it. Put on your best frown; really scrunch up your face and worry. Now replace that frown with a great big smile. What happened? Your head lifted along with your spirits. You have broken the gloom and doom cycle that can interfere with your effectiveness simply by smiling.

When you are driving and feeling pressured, smile and see what happens. It won't turn the people around you into better drivers, but you will feel more optimistic and relaxed.

Practice this technique. Use it frequently. Get in touch with the changes you can make in your outlook and attitude just by smiling. And when you are feeling that uncomfortable stress during the NCLEX, put a smile on your face and focus on the relief you feel. This simple act will free up your mind to concentrate on the questions at hand.

Breathing: You have to do it, so why not do it right?

Many Eastern cultures believe that breathing is soul-lifting, while we in the West take breathing for granted and ignore the immense benefits it offers. As a stress management technique, breathing should be right at the top of your list of ways to get through a stressful experience.

Chapter 17: Take a deep breath

Western cultures usually place the most emphasis on inhalation. Remember what you learned in nursing school about assessing your patient's breathing? Much of the emphasis was placed on inspiration, which was considered "the beginning" of respiration. Many Eastern cultures believe that good breathing begins with exhalation and that emptying the lungs of as much air as possible is the essence of healthy/healing breathing.

Advocates for conscious breathing teach and advocate breathing as a way to gain control of the sympathetic nervous system to diminish its negative effects on the cardiovascular system. When we focus on slowing our breathing, we are opposing the sympathetic nervous system's hurry-up mode and allowing the slowing of the parasympathetic nervous system to gain more control.

Let's face it, you're going to be breathing throughout the NCLEX, so you may as well make the most of it and develop a breathing technique that will work to your benefit.

Breathing under stress

When you are under stress, your breaths become shallow and rapid. Your response to stressful questions is similar to the "fight or flight" response when you are in danger. Yes, when you are running away from a lion you need the response that is mediated by the sympathetic nervous system. But when you are studying, you want your breathing to be well modulated so that adequate oxygen is getting to the cells of your body. You want to be able to think through your ideas, use those critical-thinking skills, and solve the problem at hand.

Pay attention to how you are breathing when you are faced with a difficult question. A simple start is to get control of your breathing to calm your body and mind. Remember this technique when you are sitting in the exam room taking the NCLEX.

Take a deep breath . . .

Those of you who practice yoga will already be familiar with the benefits of breathing deeply and more regularly. Filling your lungs completely dissipates tiredness and restores your mental balance. So, take advantage of this free brain refresher. After all, you always have it with you.

Take a deep breath — Chapter 17

 **Tip:** Here's a technique you can use to beat the stress and relax.

> ## Breathing to relieve stress
>
> Exhale completely.
> Expand your abdomen as you inhale deeply.
> Expand your chest as you continue to inhale.
> Now keep inhaling as your shoulders rise.
> Hold the breath for a few seconds.
> Exhale by relaxing your shoulders.
> Continue to exhale while you relax your chest.
> Exhale while you contract your abdomen.
> Repeat this exercise several times.

Don't wait until you are taking the test to practice this breathing sequence. Practice it frequently as you prepare for the NCLEX. Breathing will open your mind to learning and focusing on your study material. Remember to exhale completely and quietly; your breathing should not be audible. You can use this simple technique whenever you need it during the test. And it will come in handy as you practice nursing and deal with stressful nursing situations.

It's good for you, too

An added bonus to conscious breathing is weight loss! Yes, it's true: Healthy breathing causes your body to use oxygen more efficiently and improves your metabolism. So, studying for the NCLEX has some unforeseen bonuses, especially if you focus on improving your breathing so that you are filling and emptying your lungs more completely. Healthy breathing leads to more efficient body metabolism, reduces food cravings, increases energy, and controls weight.

Chapter 17

Take a deep breath

> "When I was studying, I got so scared that I was not going to pass that I made myself go walk on the beach, then just sit breathing, calmly enjoying the breeze and sound of the water. It really helped me feel better."
>
> —P.M., newly-practicing RN
>
> "When I get stressed, I find I get angry easily. That made everything worse, especially with my family. So when I was studying, I really worked on taking a positive view and relaxing. Sometimes I watched comedy shows on TV because laughing and smiling felt good."
>
> —R.G., successful RN
>
> "I found I got stressed when I studied alone for too long, so I called classmates to set up a study session. That really helped me."
>
> —N.D., passed NCLEX the first time

Chapter 18

Exercise your stress away

The merit badge of exercise

The preceding chapter talked about efficient breathing and energy, so now let's talk about the benefits of exercise. Right now you're probably thinking, "I'm too busy studying for the NCLEX to go to the gym or exercise. It takes too much time." But what if you knew how much more efficient your study time could be if you were at the peak of your study game every time you sat down with book in hand?

Exercise rejuvenates the body and the mind. A simple 30-minute walk has beneficial effects. Physiologically, walking provides aerobic exercise to boost your mood, and the endorphins released help relieve pain while they create a sense of well-being. This helps reduce your stress, as well as preparing your brain for studying.

Schedule your exercise

You have a study schedule, right? You know that exercise is important, so add some dedicated time for exercise to your study schedule and you will reap the rewards in improved and focused study. Take a look at the calendar on the next page for some ideas for your schedule.

Chapter 18   Exercise your stress away

Study calendar

Monday	Tuesday	Wednesday	Thursday	Friday	Saturday	Sunday
1 Lab interpretation	**2** Growth and development 7:00 pm yoga	**3** OB post partum	**4** Legal/ethical	**5** Review nutrition	**6** Study DRUGS, esp. cardiac	**7** ? P
8 S & S Bi-polar, Schiz	**9** Pedi—NEC, PKU 7:00 pm yoga	**10** Hepatitis A, B, C 8:00 pm P	**11** Study DRUGS, esp. cardiac—NEEDS MORE WORK W	**12**	**13** W	**14** ? P
15	**16** 7:00 pm yoga	**17** W	**18**	**19** W	**20** Meet Deb at park	**21** ? P
22	**23** 7:00 pm yoga	**24** W	**25**	**26** W	**27**	**28** ? P
29	**30** 7:00 pm yoga	**31**				

Key: **W** = Walk 20 min
            ? = Answer at least 50 NCLEX questions
            P = Play!

If you belong to a gym, make sure you go on a regular basis. Add "gym time" to your daily planner. Consider going three times a week for 45 minutes each time, or go to three exercise classes a week, such as aerobics or Pilates.

Tip: Think about all the ways you can get exercise. You don't have to run on a treadmill to be exercising. The key is to find something you enjoy, which means you will be more likely to do it.

Do you have a bicycle, Rollerblades, or a kayak? Break them out! Pick up that old tennis racquet or set of golf clubs. The important thing is to get moving and to have fun.

In addition to the physical benefits of exercise, you will be clearing out the cobwebs in your brain, and getting ready to store more facts and use your critical-thinking skills.

> "When I got worked up studying, I went to the gym, lifted weights, and blew off that stress on the StairMaster."
>
> —B.R., recent NCLEX taker
>
> "I took some taped lessons to the gym and listened while I was on the treadmill. I killed two birds with one stone and didn't feel like I was isolated and stuck studying!"
>
> —G.B., recent NCLEX taker

Find a buddy

Exercising regularly is easier if you have a buddy to do it with you. Ask a friend or classmate if he or she wants to join you as you exercise. You may even be able to team up with a regular at your gym.

Don't be shy. Many exercisers would love to have a workout buddy to motivate them. The support of another person means you are likely to stick with the exercise program and you will probably have more fun.

Chapter 18 — Exercise your stress away

You put one foot in front of the other

Walking as few as 10 minutes a day can benefit you and your NCLEX quest. During exercise your breathing becomes more regular and deeper, which sends oxygen to all the parts of your body. We've already discussed the benefits of breathing deeply and efficiently—walking helps you do that.

Fact: Walking is simple, cheap, and easy. You can even do it in your living room or bedroom if the weather is inclement or you don't have a safe place to walk.

The benefits of walking

Reduces stress
Clears your mind
Gives you an opportunity to tap into your creative side
Helps you generate new ideas
Lets you solve your problems on foot

Maybe some of your graduating classmates will be interested in forming a walking group. Try to walk at least three times a week for about 20 minutes each time. You may want to use this walking time just to "smell the roses" and relax. The important thing to remember is that exercise rids your body of stress, improves sleep patterns, and improves breathing.

Walking and listening

While you are walking consider listening to soothing music or inspirational-message tapes that will put you in a positive frame of mind. Check out the Internet for inspirational and positive messages.

Or you may want to combine walking with studying. During your walking time you could listen to recorded NCLEX questions or listen to those old lectures you recorded during nursing school. Check out your local bookstore for a supply of NCLEX tapes or CDs—you can even use them with your iPod.

Regardless of whether you turn walking into learning or just use it to blow off stress and increase your endorphins, get some exercise. It will improve your outlook and energy pattern. Think of exercise as mandatory, not optional.

Balance your body with yoga

Yoga has long been regarded as one of the ultimate stress relievers, meaning that now is the ideal time to take it up. Yoga is seen as both a means to physical health and a way to spiritual mastery. There are many different forms of yoga and serious students of yoga extol one form over another. However, if you want to use yoga as a relaxation tool as you prepare for the NCLEX, all you need to know is that you should pick a yoga class that works for you. As well as dedicated yoga studios, many gyms and YMCAs offer classes.

Yoga consists of a series of movements designed to integrate the body, the mind, and the spirit. Breathing is integral to performing yoga, as are stretching and achieving certain poses that are seen as ways of connecting to and being mindful of the total body. One of the key benefits attributed to yoga is stabilization of the autonomic nervous system. Remember the sympathetic and parasympathetic systems that speed up and slow down body responses and functions?

The stretching and breathing in yoga slow down the body and create an internal peacefulness. Your body feels refreshed, your circulation is improved, and your immune system gets a boost. Furthermore, yoga helps center your attention and increases your ability to concentrate. Being able to concentrate and center your attention will be extremely beneficial as you take the NCLEX.

Yoga movements incorporate the benefits of conscious breathing, which we discussed in the preceding chapter. You may want to play soothing music while performing yoga movements. The entire experience can serve to refresh and energize.

Try to find a buddy with whom to do yoga. You'll be more likely to stick to the classes and will have the added benefit of spending time with a friend. You may discover that you want to continue practicing yoga throughout your nursing career because it helps to keep your mental status at peak performance and your muscles strong.

What about tai chi?

Tai chi is sometimes called *moving meditation*. Although it is considered a martial art, most people do tai chi to improve balance, reduce stress, and enhance health. The meditative benefits of tai chi improve mental functioning and sharpen thought processes. You may hear the phrase "increasing the elasticity of the mind" when someone describes tai chi.

Tai chi involves a series of movements designed to occur over the individual's center of gravity. Some Eastern cultures recommend tai chi as part of the routine treatment plan for many illnesses and conditions. The energy the body releases when practicing tai chi alters physical and mental awareness and helps to increase mindfulness and self-direction.

In Chinese medicine, practitioners believe tai chi frees the flow of qi (pronounced "chee") in the body. Qi is believed to be the essence of health and wellness. Although qi is an unfamiliar concept for many Westerners, physicians in this country are increasingly recommending tai chi for patients with a variety of physical conditions. There is strong evidence that the practice of tai chi dramatically improves balance and increases muscle strength.

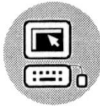

Click: A great deal of information about the benefits of tai chi is available on the Internet. For a simple discussion of tai chi and its benefits (and yoga and other stress relievers), visit the Helpguide site, at *www.helpguide.org/mental/stress_relief_meditation_yoga_relaxation.htm*.

The National Center for Complementary and Alternative Medicine, part of the National Institutes of Health, has a useful article on tai chi at *http://nccam.nih.gov/health/taichi*.

Consider trying tai chi as a relaxation and mind-strengthening technique. Classes are readily available, are usually inexpensive, and require no special equipment. Tai chi is also something you can practice easily at home.

Exercise without even noticing

The benefits of exercise are so important that you should take any opportunity you can to squeeze some in and improve your studying. There are many easy ways to exercise without really noticing you're doing it.

Exercise your stress away — Chapter 18

Exercise without exercising

Here are some simple ways to exercise while doing something else:

- Use a couple of cans of ravioli as weights to lift while reading. Doing a few reps with each arm will increase circulation and tone your arms at the same time.

- If you're reading while lying on your bed or sofa, try a few stomach crunches.

- While you're sitting at your computer, squeeze your abdominal and gluteal muscles, hold them for a few seconds, and then release. This is something you can do all day long while sitting in a chair.

- Try exercising your calves while sitting at your desk. Lift your legs up on the balls of your feet and set them down. Keep doing this until your legs are comfortably tired. Then repeat again about 10 minutes later. Do this whole routine for about an hour or so to exercise your calves.

- While you're brushing your teeth in the morning, try some squats. (It's best not to do this at night because exercising right before you go to bed can make it tough to drop off to sleep.)

- Turn on the radio and dance around while vacuuming (when the dust bunnies have grown so numerous that you can't put off cleaning in favor of studying any longer).

These simple tips will help you feel energized. As an added bonus, you will also know that you have done something good for yourself.

Chapter 19

Manage stress by living well

Along with breathing techniques and regular exercise, there are other things you can do in your life to minimize your stress and maximize your readiness for sitting for the NCLEX.

Meditation

Yoga, tai chi, and breathing exercises are linked in that they focus on relieving the body of stress and increasing mindfulness. Another way of doing this is through meditation. Studies of meditation in college students reveal that those who meditate get better grades, increase their IQ, improve their memory, learn quickly, and expand the amount of their brain that is responding to stimuli.

After reading this, you are probably wondering why you didn't start meditating when you started nursing school! Well, it's not too late. Those who practice meditation on a regular basis say they experienced the benefits almost immediately after starting to meditate. They feel more alert, are better able to analyze information, and are able to remain calm, creative, and focused even in the midst of relative chaos. Further benefits include increased self-confidence, improved sleep patterns, and markedly reduced feelings of stress.

Anyone can meditate

Meditation can be learned quickly, can be practiced anywhere, and is completely free.

> **Simple meditation techniques**
>
> - Get in a comfortable position, in a place where you will not be disturbed, and sit quietly.
>
> - Pick a word or short phrase (known as a "mantra") on which to focus. You can even concentrate on your breathing.
>
> - Close your eyes.
>
> - Breathe in and out slowly as you concentrate on repeating your focus word or phrase, or listen to the sound of your breath.
>
> - Let your mind quiet as you repeat your mantra.
>
> - Don't worry if your mind wanders. Just bring yourself back to your word, phrase, or breath.
>
> - Continue for about 20 minutes.
>
> - Remain sitting for a minute or two after your 20 minutes are over.

Many people recommend meditating twice a day, but you will still derive benefits if you can do it only once a day. Before breakfast or dinner is a good time for meditation.

Click: Most bookstores have a plethora of CDs, tapes, and books on how to meditate. Many of the breathing techniques mentioned earlier in this book are part of meditation preparation. Free, guided meditations are available at *www.beliefnet.com*.

Talk to your classmates. Don't be surprised if the ones who did best on tests and seemed in control of any situation are already meditation practitioners.

Once again, this is a simple, free technique for reducing stress in preparation for the NCLEX and your nursing career. Try it! Don't get discouraged if your mind wanders. Just bring yourself back to your breath or the phrase you are using and continue. Just a little practice will bring peaceful, calming rewards.

Go to your happy place

Some people consider it a "poor man's meditation," but identifying a place where you feel safe, serene, happy, and relaxed can serve you during the NCLEX. Perhaps you feel best at the beach with the sound of the water hitting the shore. Or maybe you are a sailor and love the feel of the wind on your face as the boat cuts through the water. Or your happy place could be remembering how you felt when you first met your significant other.

Figure out whatever memory makes you feel happy and safe, and bring it to mind when you are feeling tense. This is an easy way to bring quick comfort. Try it when studying so that you have it on hand to use during the test.

> *"Thinking about my kids always brings a smile to my face. They make me happy, so I think about them—especially when I get nervous."*
>
> —T.W., recent NCLEX taker
>
> *"I play the piano when I get too bogged down with nursing. It was a great help during school and I used it for stress relief when I was studying for NCLEX."*
>
> —D.H., recent NCLEX taker

Eat for the NCLEX

Poor nutrition can cause stress. When you are getting ready to take the NCLEX, you do not want to add to your stress by eating a non-nutritious diet. Good nutrition enhances your immune system and will increase your chances of being in top form when you take the NCLEX.

Chapter 19   **Manage stress by living well**

Watch out: Experts recommend that you *not* skip meals, so make sure you don't get so engrossed in your study schedule that you forget about meal time. You should take time to eat nutritious food at least three times a day. Choose some protein, complex carbohydrates, and a little fat, and limit or eliminate simple sugars. Remember adrenal physiology? When we are stressed, we put out cortisol, which increases our cravings for sugar, fat, and salt.

Avoid munching on the wrong snacks and avoid those high-calorie junk foods. Instead, keep healthy snacks such as nuts, yogurt, fruit, string cheese, or low-fat granola on hand. Limit yourself to one or two snacks a day—don't spend all day grazing.

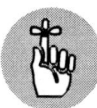

Don't forget: Remember that high-calorie snacks such as potato chips and candy bars cause your insulin levels to fluctuate widely and often leave you feeling tired, irritable, and not at the top of your game.

Tips for healthy eating

What can you do to maximize your nutritional status? Numerous Web sites provide more in-depth information on eating well and eating to reduce stress:

- The United States Department of Agriculture offers a site where you can enter your age, gender, and activity level and get information on recommended diet: *www.mypyramid.gov*.

- Check out this short nutrition survival guide from the University of North Carolina's Campus Health services: *http://shs.unc.edu/chsb/fitness_nutrition/nutrition_survivalguide.html*.

- McGill University's Student Health Services offers a quick guide to stress and nutrition: *www.mcgill.ca/studenthealth/information/nutritionalhealth/stress*.

These will get you started, but you can also go to Google and type in "stress and nutrition" to find more sites. Don't forget that your school library and state department of agriculture are also good resources for nutrition advice.

Avoid caffeine, alcohol, and cigarettes

You may think caffeine will help you stay awake to study, but caffeine is self-defeating. You may find your consumption of caffeine is contributing to your nervousness, insomnia, and headaches.

Avoid caffeinated drinks—water is the best alternative and won't give you any unpleasant side effects. Another choice is decaffeinated tea, especially green tea, which has been shown to improve your immune system.

We can't avoid mentioning alcohol and cigarettes. Don't succumb to the myth that alcohol and cigarettes are necessary to manage your stress.

Alcohol is a depressant. In small or even moderate amounts, you will enjoy some relaxation effects. If you overdo it, however, you may be left feeling depressed, more worried, and less able to manage your feelings. A word to the wise is *moderation*. Don't overdo your drinking in an effort to relax after a heavy study session. Instead, take a walk, get some fresh air, or chat with friends to unwind after studying.

Also pay attention to your smoking. Remember that the carbon monoxide in smoke takes up valuable space on your hemoglobin, meaning less oxygen gets to your brain cells. On the other hand, getting ready for the NCLEX is not the optimal time to quit smoking. Most smokers feel anxious when they try to quit, so it is best to not add to your anxiety at this time.

Moderation is the key. Think about it—maybe you can cut down or at least not go completely wild. Make a pledge to yourself and your health to quit smoking as soon as the NCLEX is over.

Don't let others drag you down

The final key to managing your stress is to stay away from naysayers. Negative thinking is contagious, but so is positive thinking. Choose to fill your physical and internal environments with positive-thinking individuals and energy.

Are you a naysayer yourself? Are you bringing yourself down with your own negativity? To find out, do a self-assessment. Consider whether you are an optimist. Can you picture getting the NCLEX results that confirm that you passed? Do you imagine yourself as an RN working in your dream job? If you are naturally optimistic, great; now is the time to consciously promote your optimistic nature. Think about ways to feed your optimism by listening to positive messages and telling yourself that you will be successful with the NCLEX.

If you tend to be pessimistic, explore the world of positive thinking. Books and audio CDs are available that can help lift your thinking. Consider reading books or listening to CDs by Zig Ziglar, Anthony Robbins, or another positive, inspirational person. This is the time to really focus on developing a positive attitude. Researchers find that people with positive attitudes think more constructively and creatively, and have an expectation of success. Visualize yourself as an RN, working at your dream job, enjoying your success. Tell yourself, "I can do this," "I am able," "I will succeed," or another inspirational message that you find promotes your positive outlook.

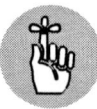

Don't forget: Many people believe that attitude equals outcome. If they are right, now is the time to develop and use a positive attitude to be successful on the NCLEX.

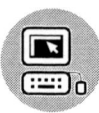

Click: The Web is full of sites about positive attitudes. One such site is *www.successconsciousness.com*. This site will lead you to many others, where you will have opportunities to test yourself and find out whether you are pessimistic.

Just say no

You may need to organize your environment by learning to say no to people who are interrupting your study schedule. Studying can be a drag and friends will want to rescue you from the boredom. You have a choice: Relinquish your study plan and go play, or remain focused on your goal to pass the NCLEX.

Don't forget to enjoy yourself

You do not have to study every minute of every day. Remember that all work and no play makes Jack a dull boy. You need to incorporate time for fun and relaxation in your schedule so that you have a chance to decompress and return to your studying refreshed and ready to learn.

When you developed your study schedule, did you include time for play and relaxation? You should have! Enlist your friends to help you stick with your study plan and to be there when your studying is over and it's time to play.

Manage stress by living well — Chapter 19

And when you play, play hard! Don't be consumed with guilt thinking you should be studying every minute. You deserve some fun and the stimulation will make it easier to concentrate when you get back to studying.

Your family and friends probably feel like they have been sacrificing, too. They have supported you through nursing school and your long study periods, and they will appreciate an hour or two to spend some time with you.

Make the most of your free time

Here are some suggestions for things to do for fun:

- Hang out with family or friends.
- Go to the playground with kids (either your own or borrowed).
- Catch a movie.
- Sing karaoke.
- Treat yourself to a manicure.
- Take a long bubble bath.
- Play with your dog.
- Get a massage.
- Play sports with a friend.
- Do something creative, such as painting a picture, working on a scrapbook, or playing an instrument.
- Play a board game.
- Jump rope.

Take time to do something that makes you laugh and gives you a genuine break from studying and thinking about the NCLEX. Give yourself some positive feedback that you deserve to feel happy and be successful on the NCLEX.

Chapter 20

The big day

It's finally here: the big day you have been preparing for and stressing about for weeks, if not since your very first day in nursing school. And guess what—you woke up this morning and suddenly found you could not remember a single thing you ever learned in nursing school.

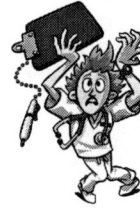

Don't panic: Take a deep breath and calm down. You have all the tools you need to be successful. You made it through nursing school and you created a sensible study schedule that has prepared you to tackle the test with confidence.

You are bound to have a few butterflies on test day—remember that some stress is a good thing—and the techniques you have already learned to combat stress will come in handy on this important day.

Chapter 20: The big day

> ### Before you sit for the test
>
> - Be prepared; study thoroughly.
>
> - Wear comfortable clothing.
>
> - Take a dry run to the location prior to test day so that you do not get lost.
>
> - Allow plenty of time to arrive.
>
> - Get everything you need to take with you out and ready to go the night before.
>
> - Ensure that you have the proper ID with you.
>
> - Don't forget your Authorization to Test (sit pass).
>
> - Breathe and smile.
>
> - Keep telling yourself: "I can do this."

Relaxation techniques for the NCLEX

The techniques we have already talked about will be useful on test day. Smiling, breathing, and maintaining a positive attitude will be with you throughout the exam. No one but you will know that you are successfully managing your stress, so take advantage of your toolkit and use these tools as often as necessary.

Practice ahead of time when you are working your way through practice questions and you feel tension building. Take some deep breaths, smile, and tell yourself, "I can do this."

During the test

Sitting in a quiet room to take the test can be an unnerving experience, but take advantage of the quiet and clear your mind. Take a minute or two and breathe deeply, clearing your mind of all distraction so that you can focus on the task at hand.

Don't let time stress you out. Remember when you worked on the practice questions and set a timer? You know how long a minute really is, and you know you have a surprisingly long time to dissect a question and figure out the best response.

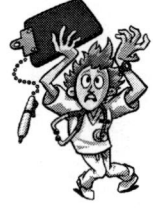

Don't panic: Do not let a fear of the clock cause you to rush through the test. Make sure you read the questions thoroughly and think about your answers using your critical-thinking skills.

Another thing that may cause some stress is the person who will be walking around the room and looking over your shoulder. Do not be freaked out by the monitor, who is there to ensure that the test is taken fairly. This is when your techniques for increasing your focus will come in handy. Think about the monitor being in the room before you go in so that you are not unnerved when he or she walks behind you.

What worried you?

> "I was so worried about time and felt as though I would run out of time before I finished the exam. Then I was amazed at how much time I ended up having and I finished the exam with plenty of time to spare. Afterward, I wished I had practiced timing myself—it would have saved lots of worry during the exam."
>
> —K.M., successful NCLEX taker
>
> "I didn't think beforehand about having the monitor looking over my shoulder. It interfered with my concentration because I wasn't prepared."
>
> —J.L., passed despite being unnerved

Chapter 20   **The big day**

What if I'm taking the test and I hit a snag?

Let's say you are making progress on the NCLEX and are working your way through the questions, but you come across a question such as this:

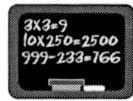

Example: Which assessment finding would you expect in a 16-year-old boy with Hodgkin's lymphoma?

When you get a question such as this, you may panic because you know very little about Hodgkin's disease. But remember: The key to NCLEX success is not to memorize every fact. That would be impossible. NCLEX success comes from using your critical-thinking skills to work through a problem, apply your knowledge, and deduce the best answer.

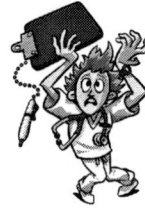

Don't panic: Take a deep breath, smile, and think about what you know about Hodgkin's disease. It has something to do with the lymph nodes and is worse if it is above and below the diaphragm, right? Take a look at the answer choices:

    a. small, tender nodes in the groin

    b. enlarged, firm, nontender nodes in the supra-clavicular area

    c. enlarged, tender nodes all over the body

    d. small, nontender, moveable nodes in the cervical area

Okay, you have studied nodes and cancer, so that is familiar. And Hodgkin's is a form of cancer of the lymph system. Can you relate this to anything about which you feel confident? Tender nodes are usually associated with inflammation or infection, so you can eliminate choices "a" and "c". Do you know anything about what it means if a node is movable or nonmovable? Yes. Typically, moveable nodes are less likely to be malignant. By using the process of elimination, your best guess is choice "b": enlarged, firm, nontender node in the supra-clavicular area. And guess what? You are right!

See how we worked through a question you thought you did not know the answer to, by using critical-thinking skills?

Let's try another one.

How about a pediatric example? A question on pediatrics may require more than one deep breath. Remember to slow down and get control of that sympathetic nervous system.

The big day — Chapter 20

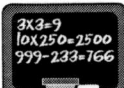

Example: What cognitive skills do you expect a 6-year-old to have?

    a. able to understand basic rules

    b. able to understand abstract concepts

    c. able to recognize object permanence

    d. able to imitate others

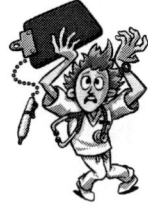

Don't panic: Stop and think. Remember your brother, cousin, neighbor, or the kid you used to baby-sit? Let's assume you can't remember anything about object permanence, but you are pretty sure that is not the right answer. You think abstract thought is for adolescents. That leaves you with two choices left to ponder. Ask yourself, do six-year-olds have to understand basic rules and follow them? Yes, they do. Six-year-olds are just starting school—school requires that children follow simple rules, such as no talking in class, staying in line while walking to the cafeteria, and so on.

So, that is the answer that makes sense, and it is a very good choice.

> "I had a question about spinal meningitis and I went blank. All could remember was my instructor saying, 'these kids are really, really sick.' So I looked for the answer that seemed like the child would be the sickest!"
>
> —T.M., recent NCLEX taker

Think about what you know

Many questions will have you looking for the answer you know is correct. But often you will be faced with a question for which you do not immediately "know" the answer. This is where you have to critically think through the options, just like we did with the two examples we just completed.

Use the same technique for questions you are unsure about and that you need to break down and sift through more slowly. The key is to focus on de-stressing yourself and thinking through what you know about the topic.

Chapter 20   **The big day**

You have learned so much in your time at nursing school. The answer will be there—you just need to stay calm and use your tools to unlock the secret.

You are ready!

So, there you have it: all the information you need to study wisely and all the tools you need to tackle the test with confidence. Do not allow yourself to be overwhelmed when you're in the test center. Just stay calm—you already have all the tools you need.

Formula for sanity and success on the NCLEX

- Take a deep breath.
- Read the question carefully.
- Be sure you know what the question is asking.
- Look for the answer you know.
- Remember to smile, breathe again, and stay calm.
- Think about what you know about the topic.
- Sift and sort through the answer choices.
- Based on your critical-thinking analysis, choose your answer.
- Move to the next question.
- Focus only on the question at hand, not on how you did on previous questions.

This is your test. You know everything you need to know to be successful. Good luck, you will be a great nurse. Welcome to the profession!

Appendix

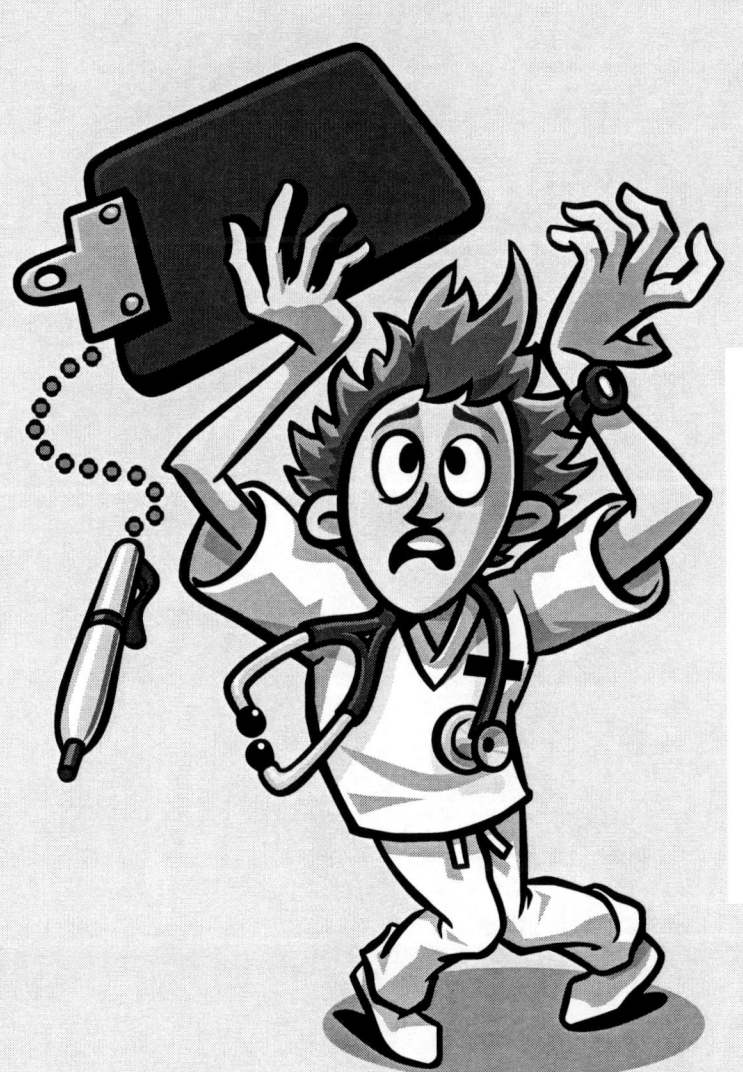

- Study guide quiz
- Resources
- Glossary
- References
- Study guide quiz answers

Study guide quiz

These questions are intended to jog your memory and make you think about the areas you need to review in your text books. Have a go and let the questions help you identify areas on which you need to spend more study time. Answers are at the back of the book.

Medications

1. What's the difference between absorption and distribution of drugs in the body?

2. Why it is important to know where drugs are metabolized?

3. What is meant by the peak and trough for some drugs?

4. How does decreased serum albumin level interact with drug toxicity?

Clinical practice

1. What are the key criteria for developing a client specific outcome objective?

2. When does the nurse initiate discharge planning?

3. Who should the nurse include when planning care for a client?

4. What guides the ethical practice of nursing?

Study guide quiz

5. What are some activities registered nurses use to evaluate and improve nursing practice?

6. What is the difference between assault and battery?

7. How could a nurse commit false imprisonment of a client?

8. What is the purpose of the Nurse Practice Act?

9. What's the difference between malpractice and negligence?

10. How would you apply Maslow's hierarchy of needs to nursing care delivery?

11. What layers of tissue are involved in a stage III pressure ulcer?

12. Which of the following patients should the nurse care for first?

    - A client who needs to get up to go to the bathroom?
    - A client with a tracheostomy who needs to be suctioned?
    - A client asking for pain medication?
    - A client who needs to be catheterized for a sterile urine specimen?

13. A patient has an ulcer that is a round, 4mm reddened area with partial thickness skin loss involving a blister. At what stage is this ulcer?

14. When opening a sterile package, should the nurse open the first flap away from or toward self?

Cardiovascular

To get you thinking—and hopefully reviewing—your textbook on cardiovascular!

1. The sinus node initiates the cardiac cycle sending an electrical impulse to the atrial node which then conveys the impulse to the _____ and finally to the _____.

2. What signs and symptoms are specific for cardiac disease?

> Study guide quiz

3. What enzymes are found after myocardial injury?

4. What finding would you expect in a patient with right ventricular failure?

5. Why is morphine given to patients with pulmonary edema?

Medical-surgical questions

These general questions are designed to help you identify areas where you need to spend some time reviewing your textbooks.

1. Your patient requires blood transfusions and is AB+. Which type of blood can he or she receive?

2. What is the most important action the nurse must take when blood administration is ordered for a patient?

3. Why would a patient be given a Schilling test?

4. When reviewing your patient's chart, you find that his platelets and white blood cells are low. What precautions would you immediately want to include in your nursing plan of care?

5. If your patient has a chest tube to suction, you must watch for bubbling in which part of the drainage system?

6. If the alarm on your ventilated patient goes off, what should you do first? Call the physician or assess the patient?

7. Why is it important to limit/monitor the amount of oxygen given to a patient with chronic obstructive pulmonary disease (COPD)?

8. What sort of isolation is used for a patient with tuberculosis?

9. What signs and symptoms would you expect in a patient with suspected ARDS?

10. How might a patient with colon cancer describe his or her stools?

Study guide quiz

11. What dietary suggestions would you make to your patient who has just undergone gastric surgery?

12. Why is it necessary to monitor the breath sounds in a patient being treated with a Sengstaken-Blakemore tube to tamponade esophageal varices?

13. What are the differences in the way Hepatitis A and B are transmitted?

14. How much drainage from the T-tube should the nurse expect from a patient who had an abdominal cholecystectomy with T-tube placement?

Resources

The following pages list resources and organizations that may be helpful to you. All contact information is current as of the date of publication.

NCLEX information

National Council of State
Boards of Nursing
NCLEX Examinations Department
111 East Wacker Drive, Suite 2900
Chicago, IL 60601-4277
Phone: (866) 293-9600
www.ncsbn.org

NCLEX Examination Program
Pearson Professional Testing
5601 Green Valley Drive
Bloomington, MN 55437-1099
Phone: (866) 49NCLEX
(or 866/496-1539)
www.pearsonvue.com/nclex

State Boards of Nursing

Alabama Board of Nursing
770 Washington Avenue
RSA Plaza, Suite 250
P.O. Box 303900
Montgomery, AL 36130-3900
Phone: (334) 242-4060
www.abn.state.al.us

Alaska Board of Nursing
Department of Comm. & Econ. Development
Division of Occupational Licensing
550 W. 7th Avenue, Suite 1500
Anchorage, AK 99501-3567
Phone: (907) 269-8161
www.dced.state.ak.us/occ/pnur.htm

American Samoa Health Services
Services Regulatory Board
LBJ Tropical Medical Center
Pago Pago, AS 96799
Phone: (684) 633-1222

Arizona State Board of Nursing
4747 N. 7th Street, Suite 200
Phoenix, AZ 85014
Phone: (602) 889-5150
www.azbn.gov

Arkansas State Board of Nursing
University Tower Building
1123 S. University, Suite 800
Little Rock, AR 72204-1619
Phone: (501) 686-2700
www.arsbn.org

Resources

California Board of Registered Nursing
1625 North Market Boulevard
Suite N217
Sacramento, CA 95834
Phone: (916) 322-3350
www.rn.ca.gov

California Board of Vocational Nurse
and Psychiatric Technician Examiners
2535 Capitol Oaks Drive, Suite 205
Sacramento, CA 95833
Phone: (916) 263-7800
www.bvnpt.ca.gov

Colorado Board of Nursing
1560 Broadway, Suite 880
Denver, CO 80202
Phone: (303) 894-2430
www.dora.state.co.us/nursing

Connecticut Board of Examiners
for Nursing
Department of Public Health
410 Capitol Avenue, MS# 13PHO
P.O. Box 340308
Hartford, CT 06134-0308
Phone: (860) 509-7648
www.dph.state.ct.us

Delaware Board of Nursing
861 Silver Lake Boulevard
Cannon Building, Suite 203
Dover, DE 19904
Phone: (302) 739-4522
www.professionallicensing.state.de.us/boards/nursing/index.shtml

Florida Board of Nursing
4052 Bald Cypress Way, BINCO2
Tallahassee, FL 32399
Phone: (850) 245-4125
www.doh.state.fl.us/mqa/nursing

Georgia Board of Nursing
237 Coliseum Drive
Macon, GA 31217-3858
Phone: (478) 207-1300
www.sos.state.ga.us/plb/rn

Georgia State Board of Licensed
Practical Nurses
237 Coliseum Drive
Macon, GA 31217-3858
Phone: (912) 207-1300
www.sos.state.ga.us/plb/lpn

Guam Board of Nurse Examiners
P.O. Box 2816
Hagtana, GU 96932
Phone: (671) 735-7406

Hawaii Board of Nursing
Professional and Vocational
Licensing Division
Attention: BON
P.O. Box 3469
Honolulu, HI 96801
Phone: (808) 586-3000
www.hawaii.gov/dcca/areas/pvl/boards/nursing

Idaho Board of Nursing
280 N. 8th Street, Suite 210
P.O. Box 83720
Boise, ID 83720-0061
Phone: (208) 334-3110
www.state.id.us/ibn

Illinois Department of
Professional Regulation
James R. Thompson Center
100 West Randolph, Suite 9-300
Chicago, IL 60601
Phone: (312) 814-2715
www.idfpr.com

Resources

Indiana State Board of Nursing
Professional Licensing Agency
402 W. Washington Street
Room W072
Indianapolis, IN 46204
Phone: (317) 234-2043
www.in.gov/pla

Iowa Board of Nursing
RiverPoint Business Park
400 S.W. 8th Street, Suite B
Des Moines, IA 50309-4685
Phone: (515) 281-3255
www.state.ia.us/government/nursing

Kansas State Board of Nursing
Landon State Office Building
900 S.W. Jackson Street, Suite 1051
Topeka, KS 66612-1230
Phone: (785) 296-4929
www.ksbn.org

Kentucky Board of Nursing
312 Whittington Parkway, Suite 300
Louisville, KY 40222
Phone: (502) 429-3300
www.kbn.ky.gov

Louisiana State Board of
Practical Nurse Examiners
3421 N. Causeway Boulevard
Suite 505
Metairie, LA 70002
Phone: (504) 838-5791
www.lsbpne.com

Louisiana State Board of Nursing
5207 Essen Lane, Suite 6
Baton Rogue, LA 70809
Phone: (225) 763-3570
www.lsbn.state.la.us

Maine State Board of Nursing
158 State House Station
Augusta, ME 04333-0158
Phone: (207) 287-1133
www.maine.gov/bon

Maryland Board of Nursing
4140 Patterson Avenue
Baltimore, MD 21215-2254
Phone: (410) 585-1900
www.mbon.org

Massachusetts Board of Registration
in Nursing
Commonwealth of Massachusetts
239 Causeway Street, Second Floor
Boston, MA 02114
Phone: (617) 973-0800
www.mass.gov/dpl/boards/htm

Michigan Bureau of
Health Professions
Ottawa Building
611 W. Ottawa Street, 1st Floor
Lansing, MI 48933
Phone: (517) 8068
www.michigan.gov/healthlicense

Minnesota Board of Nursing
2829 University Avenue SE, Suite 200
Minneapolis, MN 55414
Phone: (612) 617-2270
www.nursingboard.state.mn.us

Mississippi Board of Nursing
1935 Lakeland Drive, Suite B
Jackson, MS 39216
Phone: (601) 944-4826
www.msbn.state.ms.us

Resources

Missouri State Board of Nursing
3605 Missouri Boulevard
P.O. Box 656
Jefferson City, MO 65102-0656
Phone: (573) 751-0681
http://pr.mo.gov/nursing/asp

Montana State Board of Nursing
301 South Park
P.O. Box 200513
Helena, MT 59620-0513
Phone: (406) 841-2340
www.mt.gov

Nebraska Department of Health
and Human Services
Department of Regulation and Licensure
Nursing Section
301 Centennial Mall South
Lincoln, NE 68509-5007
Phone: (402) 471-4376
www.hhs.state.ne.us

New Hampshire Board of Nursing
21 South Fruit Street, Suite 16
Concord, NH 03301
Phone: (603) 271-2323
www.state.nh.us/nursing

New Jersey Board of Nursing
P.O. Box 45010
124 Halsey Street, 6th Floor
Newark, NJ 07101
Phone: (973) 504-6430
www.state.nj.us/lps/ca/medical/nursing.htm

New Mexico Board of Nursing
6301 Indian School Road, NE
Suite 710
Albuquerque, NM 87110
Phone: (505) 841-8340
www.bon.state.nm.us/index/html

New York State Education Department
Office of the Professions
State Board for Nursing
89 Washington Avenue
Albany, NY 12234
Phone: (518) 474-3817, Ext. 120
www.op.nysed.gov/nurse.htm

North Carolina Board of Nursing
3724 National Drive Camden Building
Suite 201
Raleigh, NC 27612
Phone: (919) 782-3211
www.ncbon.com

North Dakota Board of Nursing
919 South 7th Street, Suite 504
Bismark, ND 58504
Phone: (701) 328-9777
www.ndbon.org

Ohio Board of Nursing
17 South High Street, Suite 400
Columbus, OH 43215-7410
Phone: (614) 466-3947
www.nursing.ohio.gov

Oklahoma Board of Nursing
2915 N. Classen Boulevard,
Suite 524
Oklahoma City, OK 73106
Phone: (405) 962-1800
www.ok.gov/nursing

Oregon State Board of Nursing
800 Oregon Street NE, Suite 465
Portland, OR 97232-2162
Phone: (971) 673-0685
www.oregon.gov/OSBN

Resources

Commonwealth of Puerto Rico
Board of Nurse Examiners
800 Roberto H. Todd Avenue
Room 202, Stop 18
Santurce, PR 00908
Phone: (787) 725-7506
www.nurse.org/pr-index.shtml

Pennsylvania State Board of Nursing
P.O. Box 2649
Harrisburg, PA 17105-2649
Phone: (717) 783-7142
www.dos.state.pa.us/nurse

Rhode Island Board of Nurse
Registration and Nursing Education
Three Capitol Hill, Room 105
Providence, RI 02908
Phone: (401) 222-5700
*www.health.state.ri/us/hsr/
professions/nurses.php*

South Carolina State Board of Nursing
Synergy Business Park
Kingstree Building
110 Centerview Drive, Suite 202
Columbia, SC 29210
Phone: (803) 896-4550
www.llr.state.sc.us/pol/nursing

South Dakota Board of Nursing
4305 South Louise Ave., Suite 201
Sioux Falls, SD 57106-3115
Phone: (605) 362-2760
www.state.sd.us/doh/nursing

Tennessee State Board of Nursing
227 French Landing Suite 300
Nashville, TN 37243
Phone: (615) 532-3202
www2.state.tn.us/health/boards/nursing

Texas Board of Nurse Examiners
333 Guadalupe, Suite 3-460
Austin, TX 78701
Phone: (512) 305-7400
www.bne.state.tx.us

Utah State Board of Nursing
Heber M. Wells Building, 4th Floor
160 East 300 South
Salt Lake City, UT 84111
Phone: (801) 530-6628
www.dopl.utah.gov/licensing/nurse.html

Vermont State Board of Nursing
81 River Street
Montpelier, VT 05609-1106
Phone: (802) 828-2396
www.vtprofessionals.org/nurses

Virgin Islands Board of
Nurse Licensure
Veterans Drive Station
P.O. Box 4247
St. Thomas, VI 00803
Phone: (340) 776-7397

Virginia Board of Nursing
6603 W. Broad Street, 5th Floor
Richmond, VA 23230-1712
Phone: (804) 662-9909
www.dhp.virginia.gov/nursing

Washington State Nursing
Care Quality
Assurance Commission
Department of Health
310 Israel Road
Turnwater, WA 98501
Phone: (360) 236-4700
*https://fortress.wa.gov/doh/hpqa1/hps6/
Nursing/default.htm*

Resources

West Virginia State Board of Examiners
for Licensed Practical Nurses
101 Dee Drive
Charleston, WV 25311
Phone: (304) 558-3572
www.lpnboard.state.wv.us

West Virginia Board of Examiners
for Registered Professional Nurses
101 Dee Drive, Suite 102
Charleston, WV 25311
Phone: (304) 558-3596
www.wvrnboard.com

Wisconsin Department of Regulation
and Licensing
1400 E. Washington Avenue
P.O. Box 8935
Madison, WI 53708-8935
Phone: (608) 266-2112
http://drl.wi.gov/boards/nur

Wyoming State Board of Nursing
1810 Pioneer Avenue
Cheyenne, WY 82002
Phone: (307) 777-7601
http://nursing.state.wy.us

Student organizations

Chi Eta Phi Student Nurse Sorority
3029 13th Street, NW
Washington, DC 20009
Phone: (202) 232-3858
www.chietaphi.com

National Student Nurses' Association
45 Main Street, Suite 606
Brooklyn, NY 11201
Phone: (718) 210-0705
www.nsna.org

Sigma Theta Tau International
Honor Society of Nursing
550 W. North Street
Indianapolis, IN 46202
Phone: (317) 634-8171
www.nursingsociety.org

National Organization for Associate
Degree Nursing
7794 Grow Drive
Pensacola, FL 32514
Phone: (850) 484-6948
www.noadn.org

Professional Associations

American Assembly for Men
in Nursing
P.O. Box 130220
Birmingham, AL 35213
Attention: Byron McCain
Phone: (205) 802-7551
www.aamn.org

American Nurses Association
8515 Georgia Avenue, Suite 400
Silver Spring, MD 20910
Phone: (301) 628-5000
www.nursingworld.org

Asian American & Pacific Islander
Nurses Association
252 Silleck Street
Clifton, NJ 07013
www.aapina.org

National League for Nursing
61 Broadway, 33rd Floor
New York, NY 10006
Phone: (212) 363-5555
www.nln.org

Resources

National Alaska Native/American
Indian Nurses Association
3702 S. Fife Street
Tacoma, WA 98409-7318
www.nanainanurses.org

National Association of
Hispanic Nurses
1501 16th Street, NW
Washington, DC 20036
Phone: (202) 387-2477
www.thehispanicnurses.org

National Black Nurses
Association, Inc.
8630 Fenton Street, Suite 330
Silver Spring, MD 20910-3803
Phone: (301) 589-3200
www.nbna.org

National Federation of Licensed
Practical Nurses, Inc.
605 Poole Drive
Garner, SC 27529
Phone: (919) 779-0046
www.nflpn.org

Philippine Nurses Association
of America
151 Linda Vista Drive
Daly City, CA 94014
Phone: (415) 468-7995
www.philippinenursesaa.org

Glossary

Authorization to Test (ATT) – ATT issued by Pearson VUE to allow candidates to schedule testing time and date.

Board of Nursing – Members of the board are appointed by the governor for the purpose of overseeing nurses practicing in a state. The board also has full-time employees who manage the daily operations. The board's duties include determining if license applicants are eligible, reviewing criminal background checks, managing the impaired nurses program, and revising educational requirements for student and practicing nurses.

Candidate Bulletin – Found at the National Council of State Boards of Nursing Web site (*www.ncsbn.com*) or can be requested by mail. The bulletin provides a step-by-step process for applying and taking the NCLEX.

Care plan – A written plan of action tailored specifically to patient needs. It includes nursing diagnoses and patient assessment, nursing interventions to be used, and expected outcomes.

Centers for Disease Control (CDC) – Component of the Department of Health and Human Services (HHS) responsible for protecting the health and safety of Americans.

Computer Adaptive Testing (CAT) – Computer-based examinations capable of selecting appropriate questions based on the answers provided by the test taker.

Confidentiality – A legal and ethical obligation to protect the privacy of healthcare consumers.

Glossary

Critical thinking – An organized, cognitive process for identifying underlying assumptions in various situations. A method for exploring alternatives and selecting the best approach to a problem.

Documentation – A written record of actions taken, events transpired, and facts related to the condition of a patient. This includes patient history, assessments, interventions, medications given, updates on patient condition, etc.

End-of-Program Examination (EOP) – A comprehensive test required by most schools of nursing to determine readiness to successfully take the NCLEX.

Federal Welfare-to-Work Hiring Initiative – A congressionally mandated program to assist welfare recipients in transitioning from receiving welfare to joining the workforce. Provides support for training.

Joint Commission on Accreditation of Healthcare Organizations (JCAHO) – A private company retained by healthcare organizations to determine if care provided with in the organization meets national/ JCAHO standards.

Licensure – A formal document of approval by the State Board of Nursing that is required to legally practice nursing. Licensure candidates must have graduated from an accredited nursing program and successfully passed the NCLEX exam.

Meditation – A relaxation technique used to restore calm, improve thinking, and creativity.

NCLEX – National Council Licensure Examination. Must be passed by any nurse who desires a license to practice as a registered nurse.

NCSBN – National Council of State Boards of Nursing. A collaborative group of representatives from state boards of nursing that act and counsel together on matters of common interest affecting the public safety and welfare.

Nurse Practice Acts - Laws in each state that define the scope of nursing practice. State boards of nursing oversee these statutory laws.

Glossary

Nursing interventions – Therapeutic treatments administered by nurses to positively affect the health and well-being of their patients.

Nursing process – A problem-solving process where data is gathered, analyzed, and interpreted to assist in making clinical judgments, setting goals, establishing priorities, and designing therapeutic nursing interventions.

Pearson VUE – A company focused on electronic testing for professional licensure and certification.

Pinning ceremony – Traditional nursing school ceremony wherein graduating nurses receive their nursing pin. Symbolic of initiation into the society of nurses.

Qi – In Chinese medicine believed to be the essence of health and wellness (pronounced chee).

Tai chi – Movements designed to improve balance, reduce stress, and enhance health. Sometimes called moving meditation.

Yoga – Series of movements designed to integrate body, mind, and spirit.

References

ABC of Yoga. (2006). "Health benefits of yoga—Why yoga exercise is good for you." Retrieved from *www.abc-of-yoga.com*.

Cohen, S. (2006). *Critical Thinking in the Emergency Department: Skills to Assess, Analyze, and Act.* Marblehead, MA: HCPro, Inc.

Duclos-Miller, P. (2006). *Stressed Out About Your First Year of Nursing.* Marblehead, MA: HCPro, Inc.

Help Guide: Mental Health Issues. (2006). "Stress relief: Yoga, meditation, and other relaxation techniques. Retrieved from *http://www.helpguide.org/mental/stress_relief_meditation_yoga_relaxation.htm*.

National Council of State Boards of Nursing. (2006). *2006 Candidate Bulletin.* Page 8. Available at *https://www.ncsbn.org/2006_Candidate_Bulletin.pdf*.

National Council of State Boards of Nursing. (2006). *NCLEX Statistics from NCSBN.* Available at *www.ncsbn.org*.

National Council of State Boards of Nursing. (2003). *Detailed Test Plan for the NCLEX-RN Examination.* Chicago: National Council of State Boards of Nursing, Inc.

National League for Nursing. (2006). "Executive Report." Special issue of *Shaping the Future.* Fall 2006 (11).

NCLEX Course Review. (2006). Retrieved from *www.nclexinfo.com*.

References

Study Guides and Strategies. (2006). *Dealing with Test Anxiety.* Retrieved from *www.studygs.net/tstprp8.htm*

Stress Relief Strategies. (2006). Retrieved from *www.holisticmed.com/stressfree.html.*

Study guide quiz answers

Here are the answers to the questions from page 143.

Medications

1. **What's the difference between absorption and distribution of drugs in the body?** Absorption refers to the time from when the drug is taken until the time it enters the bloodstream. Distribution refers to how soon the drug is distributed throughout the body

2. **Why it is important to know where drugs are metabolized?** Metabolism, the breakdown of chemicals to their component parts, is slowed in the very young, elderly, and individuals with liver impairments.

3. **What is meant by the peak and trough for some drugs?** Peak refers to the greatest concentration of the drug in the bloodstream and is typically measured 30 minutes after an IV dose. Trough is the lowest concentration of the drug and is typically measured 30 minutes prior to the next dose.

4. **How does decreased serum albumin level interact with drug toxicity?** Drugs bind to protein and only the unbound drug has an effect on the body. Individuals with low plasma protein, e.g., the malnourished or the elderly, have decreased albumin (protein) therefore the dosage may need to be reduced to prevent toxicity in those patients.

Study guide quiz answers

Clinical practice

1. **What are the key criteria for developing a client-specific outcome objective?**
   The objective must be measurable, criterion–based, specify a time frame for evaluation, and be relevant to the client's diagnosis and care.

2. **When does the nurse initiate discharge planning?**
   Discharge planning is initiated upon admission.

3. **Who should the nurse include when planning care for a client?**
   The client, the family, relevant members of the healthcare team, payers, and others as appropriate.

4. **What guides the ethical practice of nursing?**
   The American Nurses Association's *Code of Ethics for Nurses with Interpretive Standards*.

5. **What are some activities registered nurses use to evaluate and improve nursing practice?**
   Research, leadership, advocacy, collaboration, and responsible resource utilization are all used to evaluate and improve practice.

6. **What is the difference between assault and battery?**
   Assault refers to a physical or verbal threat. Battery refers to the unlawful touching of another without consent.

7. **How could a nurse commit false imprisonment of a client?**
   Use of confinement or restraints on a person conscious of being confined and/or harmed by the confinement.

8. **What is the purpose of the Nurse Practice Act?**
   The Nurse Practice Act provides the legal structure for the practice of licensed nurses in each state. The scope of nursing practice is defined according to license held, i.e., registered nurse, licensed nurse, advanced practice nurses, etc.

9. **What's the difference between malpractice and negligence?**
   Negligence refers to the lack of what would be considered reasonable and prudent care by a similarly licensed and experienced practitioner. Malpractice refers to negligence, misconduct, or lack of skill that results in injury or loss to the recipient.

Study guide quiz answers

10. **How would you apply Maslow's hierarchy of needs to nursing care delivery?**
    The basic physiological needs must be met before higher level needs are pursued.

11. **What layers of tissue are involved in a stage III pressure ulcer?**
    Tissues involved in a stage III ulcer include full thickness skin loss, with subcutaneous damage or necrosis. Does not extend through fascia or bone.

12. **Which of the following patients should the nurse care for first?**

    - A client who needs to get up to go to the bathroom?
    - A client with a tracheostomy who needs to be suctioned?
    - A client asking for pain medication?
    - A client who needs to be catheterized for a sterile urine specimen?

    Remember your ABCs. The airway is always first priority. Your next priority would be the client who needs to go to the bathroom—you want to prevent the client from getting up without assistance and falling. Third is the client who is requesting pain medication, and last is the client who needs to be catheterized for a specimen.

13. **A patient has an ulcer that is a round, 4mm reddened area with partial thickness skin loss involving a blister. At what stage is this ulcer?**
    Stage II pressure ulcer because of reddened area with skin breakdown.

14. **When opening a sterile package, should the nurse open the first flap away from or toward self?**
    Away from self.

Study guide quiz answers

Cardiovascular

1. The sinus node initiates the cardiac cycle sending an electrical impulse to the atrial node which then conveys the impulse to the <u>Bundle of His</u> and finally to the <u>Perkinje</u> fibers.

2. What signs and symptoms are specific for cardiac disease?
   Chest pain, dyspnea, irregular heart beat, palpitations, edema, cyanosis.

3. What enzymes are found after myocardial injury?

   - Creatine-kinase MB (CKMB, normally 0%)
   - Troponin 1, LDH 1 and 2

4. What finding would you expect in a patient with right ventricular failure?
   Jugular venous distention.

5. Why is morphine given to patients with pulmonary edema?
   Slows work of breathing, decreases anxiety, and causes vasodilitation.

Medical-surgical questions

1. Your patient requires blood transfusions and is AB+. Which type of blood can he or she receive?
   Any, this is the universal recipient (A+, A-, B+, B-, AB-, AB+, O+, O-).

2. What is the most important action the nurse must take when blood administration is ordered for a patient?
   Verify the identity of the client accurately.

3. Why would a patient be given a Schilling test?
   It is the definitive test for pernicious anemia, which is a progressive macrocytic anemia characterized by intrinsic factor deficiency.

4. When reviewing your patient's chart, you find that his platelets and white blood cells are low. What precautions would you immediately want to include in your nursing plan of care?
   Remember this rule of thumb: When platelets are low, prevent bleeding. When white blood cells (WBC) are low, prevent infection.

Study guide quiz answers

5. **If your patient has a chest tube to suction, you must watch for bubbling in which part of the drainage system?**
   The water seal section. Bubbling anywhere else means the system is not functioning properly.

6. **If the alarm on your ventilated patient goes off, what should you do first? Call the physician or assess the patient?**
   First asses the patient so you have something to tell the physician. It may be that a hose is kinked or something came loose, in which case you would not need to call the physician.

7. **Why is it important to limit/monitor the amount of oxygen given to a patient with chronic obstructive pulmonary disease (COPD)?**
   Anoxia drives breathing in the patient with COPD because the body has gradually adjusted to higher levels of carbon dioxide. Too much oxygen diminishes the drive to breathe and can result in respiratory depression and apnea.

8. **What sort of isolation is used for a patient with tuberculosis?**
   Inhalation precautions, placement in a negative pressure room to keep the bacteria from entering the hallway, and the wearing of masks.

9. **What signs and symptoms would you expect in a patient with suspected ARDS?**
   Acute respiratory distress syndrome (ARDS) is a life-threatening illness characterized by low PO^2, difficulty breathing with restlessness, and use of suprasternal and intercostal muscles for breathing.

10. **How might a patient with colon cancer describe his or her stools?**
    The patient may describe change in bowel habits with alternating constipation and diarrhea, ribbon-like stools because of tumor obstruction, or some blood on stool if tumor is low in the colon.

11. **What dietary suggestions would you make to your patient who has just undergone gastric surgery?**
    Following any gastric surgery that decreases the size of the stomach, the patient is at risk for "dumping syndrome" and should eat small meals, restrict high-sugar carbohydrates, and limit the amount of fluid taken with each meal.

Study guide quiz answers

12. **Why is it necessary to monitor the breath sounds in a patient being treated with a Sengstaken-Blakemore tube to tamponade esophageal varices?**

    The balloon tamponade created by the Sengstaken-Blakemore tube may obstruct the airway. There is also a danger of aspiration when the patient vomits blood and gastric contents.

13. **What are the differences in the way Hepatitis A and B are transmitted?**

    Hepatitis A is transmitted via hand, oral, food, or fecal routes whereas Hepatitis B is transmitted parenterally and through intimate contact.

14. **How much drainage from the T-tube should the nurse expect from a patient who had an abdominal cholecystectomy with T-tube placement?**

    Typically, the drainage is between 200ml and 500ml in the first 24 hours. Less than that may indicate an obstruction in the tube or leakage of bile into the peritoneal cavity.